"Macy and Naliboff take what most pregnancy books consider an epilogue and birth a smart, compassionate companion for parents. A must-read for anyone who finds themselves staring at a new baby and feeling like a stranger in their own body and mind."

—Abby Norman, author of *Ask Me About My Uterus*

"Whether you are in the newborn stage or years out, *Your Postpartum Body* is a thorough guide for any person who has given birth. Pelvic floor issues during pregnancy and postpartum are common but not normal, and many people are left wondering what happened to their body and how they go about healing. This comprehensive guide covers changes that occur from the feet, through the pelvic floor, and into the trunk, and provides actionable guidance to resolve common issues. Uniquely, it also covers return to sport with progressive phases of movement for Pilates, CrossFit, and running. It is a solid resource and entry point for pelvic rehabilitation."

—Amanda Olson, DPT, PRPC

"Postpartum persons need this guide for their fourth trimester. This is an excellent resource for many of the common conditions after birth not commonly discussed either by providers or amongst friends and family. Ruth and Courtney bring these issues to light, making the reader not feel alone or humiliated by these private and new concerns, and give easy-to-follow strategies to allow healing to occur."

—Melissa Collard, MD, FACOG

"In *Your Postpartum Body*, Ruth and Courtney have birthed a comprehensive and accessible roadmap to understanding and recovering your postpartum self. I couldn't recommend this book more highly!"

—Catherine Hill-Verrochi, DO, FACOG

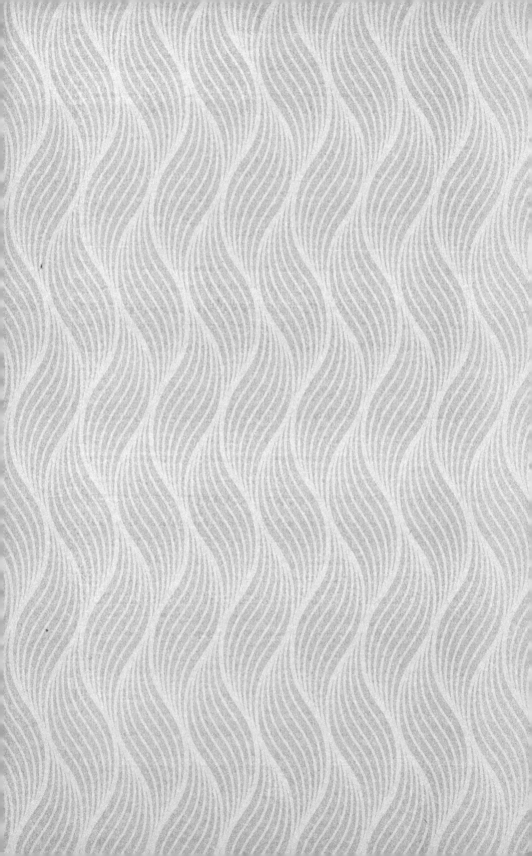

Your Postpartum Body

The Complete Guide to Healing After Pregnancy

RUTH E. MACY
PT, DPT

COURTNEY NALIBOFF

AVERY
an imprint of Penguin Random House
New York

AVERY

an imprint of Penguin Random House LLC
penguinrandomhouse.com

Photographs © William Trevaskis
Illustrations © Marie Rossettie
Title page and part opener art: Geometric wave pattern © etcberry / Shutterstock.com

Most Avery books are available at special quantity discounts for bulk purchase
for sales promotions, premiums, fundraising, and educational needs.
Special books or book excerpts also can be created to fit specific needs.
For details, write SpecialMarkets@penguinrandomhouse.com.

Library of Congress Cataloging-in-Publication Data

Names: Macy, Ruth E., author. | Naliboff, Courtney, author.
Title: Your postpartum body: the complete guide to healing
after pregnancy / Ruth E. Macy, PT, DPT, Courtney Naliboff.
Description: New York: Avery, an imprint of Penguin Random House, [2024] |
Includes index.
Identifiers: LCCN 2023044033 (print) | LCCN 2023044034 (ebook) |
ISBN 9780593541425 (trade paperback) | ISBN 9780593541432 (epub)
Subjects: LCSH: Postnatal care—Popular works. |
Postnatal exercise—Popular works.
Classification: LCC RG801.M3395 2024 (print) |
LCC RG801 (ebook) | DDC 618.6—dc23/eng/20240126
LC record available at https://lccn.loc.gov/2023044033
LC ebook record available at https://lccn.loc.gov/2023044034

Printed in the United States of America
1st Printing

Book design by Laura K. Corless

Dedicated to all those who have thought
Nobody ever told me
after pregnancy

CONTENTS

Part 1
ZERO TO SIX WEEKS POSTPARTUM

CHAPTER 1 — 3
Caring for the Postpartum Body and Mind

CHAPTER 2 — 41
Six Weeks

Contents

Part 2

HEALING THE POSTPARTUM BODY

Contents

Contents

Part 3
RETURN TO SPORT

Contents

CHAPTER 12 — 257
Yoga

CHAPTER 13 — 269
Pilates

CHAPTER 14 — 277
Running

CHAPTER 15 — 285
Kettlebell

Contents

CHAPTER 16 —— 295

CrossFit

EPILOGUE —— 301

INTRODUCTION

If you've picked up this book, chances are it's because you are looking for answers about your body. Your body is either currently growing, or at some point grew, a tiny human. During pregnancy, your body is monitored pretty closely by a team of people—nurses, midwives, doctors, maybe specialists. You might have learned some exercises you could do to prepare your body for delivery or spent a lot of the last few months in funny positions trying to get comfortable or trying to coax your body into the shape it needed to birth a human. You likely took supplements to support the tiny human's growth. You were weighed, your fundal height was measured, and your vital signs were taken regularly. You were given a lot of answers to questions you might not have even had.

But when pregnancy ends, the answers usually stop. You are considered postpartum. Very few Americans are seen more than once in their postpartum year for the health of their recovering body. You are told everything is fine. But you don't *feel* fine. You have questions about this *new* body. How long will I bleed? What can I do if breastfeeding/chestfeeding isn't going well? Are there exercises I should be doing for my core or my pelvic floor? Am I really going to leak every time I sneeze? Why is sex painful and unsatisfying?

A lot of people have these experiences, but that doesn't mean that you have to just put up with them. You, the amazing person who grew another person, have the right to know exactly what is happening to your body afterward. You have the right to know how to move, sit, exercise, have sex, and take care of yourself in ways that support the body you have now—really, the same wonderful body that you had before. You might have been told that you need to "get your body back," but guess what? You never lost it. There's just a lot to learn about it.

This book is for every postpartum human. Not all postpartum bodies are female. Not all pregnancies end in becoming a parent or with a living infant. Because of this, we have tried to use inclusive language and scenarios throughout the book. You will see *breastfeeding* also referred to as *chestfeeding*; similarly, *breast/chest/top tissue, vaginal/genital* or *front hole*, and references to the birthing person or postpartum human are used throughout the book. There may be language specific to your identity or community that isn't represented here, and we are eager to learn more inclusive and better ways to talk about the postpartum experience. All postpartum bodies go through metamorphosis, and we're here to support you through the process.

In our healthcare system, accurate information can be hard to find. Answers you receive might be based on old evidence and outdated practices, or our society at large might expect you to simply sigh and accept the fact that your body won't return to its previous function. And you may not yet know what other questions to ask.

We were just like you. Neither Ruth, who had her child in 2008, nor Courtney, who gave birth in 2014, were given education or tools, nor did we know where to turn when our bodies didn't "bounce back"— despite Ruth's career as a physical therapist, and despite the two ob-gyns in Courtney's immediate family. We were both resigned to dealing with the loss of function we experienced, because we were told this was the new normal by peers, family members, and medical professionals. But as Ruth moved into the pelvic health branch of physical therapy, she learned that although incontinence, painful intercourse, and postural adaptations are *common*, this doesn't mean they aren't *treatable*. She also learned, and helped Courtney realize, that postpartum healing isn't just possible, but a right.

We both benefited from access to postpartum healthcare, such as pelvic floor physical therapy, but we know that access is inconsistent, due to geography, availability of providers, comfort levels, or socioeconomic factors. With this book, we're giving you some practical steps you can take to support your body as it recovers from a *major* event and to promote healing even years later.

Your Postpartum Body arose from our friendship, which has lasted through moves on and off the island of North Haven, Maine, where we met; road races; paddleboarding excursions; long walks in the woods; *Star Trek* marathons; and dozens of macaroni and cheese dinners (with blueberry muffins on the side!). Ruth's expertise and Courtney's narratives will guide you through a time of your life marked by new sensations, new emotions, and new explorations of your identity. We promise you the most current research, real-life examples from postpartum humans, and some poop talk.

We have included as much evidence-based practice as we could. There are limitations in that. Science is always evolving and is limited to what is being studied and how it's being studied. In places where the science is not yet settled or robust enough, you are going to get Ruth's clinical opinion. She likes to always have an eye to what the body can do and how it can feel in the doing. There will be soft don'ts. Most medical suggestions are just that, suggestions. We recommend any soft don'ts be viewed as a "wait until," and that you always, always do what feels good for your unique body.

HOW TO USE THIS BOOK

Read this book in your second or third trimester, or at any time postpartum (even years later). Earlier in your pregnancy, you are likely focused on the pregnancy itself. Later on, your thoughts may progress toward the reality of postpartum life. We recommend reading it through at a moment when you have the time, space, and energy to do so, and then use it as a quick reference for questions, aches, dysfunctions, and concerns as they arise. The contents pages, tables, diagrams, chapter summaries, and index are all there to help you quickly navigate to the relevant parts of the book as you need them.

Part 1 leads you through the changes your body is experiencing in your fourth trimester, gives you questions to ask your medical providers, and educates you as to how to navigate the healthcare system should you need personalized healthcare that goes beyond what this book can provide. Part 2 is for when you are ready to start your physical healing. Part 3 offers specific support for returning to sports, exercise classes, and high-level fitness training. While this won't offer guidance for elite athletes, it is appropriate for anyone who finds value in sports and exercise and wants to know how to do that in a way that reduces typical postpartum symptoms.

Thank you for picking up our book. Thank you for investing in your own healing. We hope this book will give you an aha moment about your body, provide you with ways you can nurture, heal, and strengthen yourself, and empower you to advocate for yourself in a system that might seem stacked against you. So read on! Get curious about your body, all the weird things it does, and get excited to give it some loving support.

—Ruth and Courtney

Your
Postpartum
Body

Part 1

. . .

ZERO TO SIX WEEKS POSTPARTUM

So begins the journey of understanding what your body is going through immediately after delivery. Part 1 will focus on the physical and mental recovery that begins with a birth and ends with a six-week follow-up with a healthcare provider. For some of you picking up this book, zero to six weeks postpartum, or the "hazy days," are immediate. For others, this period may be months or years in the past. We highly recommend reading on if you are in the thick of it, no matter what week you are in. This is our evaluation of the aftereffects of birth, with explanations of how body, medical, cultural, and relational systems contribute to your health and healing. You will explore the changes in your body after pregnancy and cultivate three big pillars of overall health: rest, hydration, and nutrition. Read part 1, no matter what week you are postpartum, if you need to learn more about healing, navigating healthcare, caretaking your body, encouraging and discouraging lactation, or managing incisions and tears. We want to ensure that before you take off into exercise activities for healing, you do the work of managing what happened to you. Humans are complex. Healing is not linear. Experiences, and therefore needs, will vary.

IN THIS CHAPTER:

FUNCTION AND FEELING OVER APPEARANCE
   HEAD-TO-TOE POSTPARTUM BODY CHANGES
      Head
      Arms and Shoulders
      Ribs
      Breast/Chest
      Back
      Abdomen
      Pelvic Girdle
      Glutes and Legs
      Feet
      Cardiovascular
   HIERARCHY OF BODY NEEDS FOR HEALING AND RECOVERY
      Rest
      Hydration
      Nutrition
      Support

THE ROLE OF HORMONES IN POSTPARTUM RECOVERY

LACTATION AND CESSATION OF LACTATION
   BREAST MILK/HUMAN MILK: WHAT IS IT?
   ENCOURAGING LACTATION
   LACTATION: AN ISSUE OF RIGHTS AND PRIVILEGE
   SUPPORTS FOR LACTATION SUCCESS
      Education and Birthing Facility Resources
      Workplace Provisions for Pumping
      Accessories
   BREASTFEEDING/CHESTFEEDING BASICS
   LACTATION CHALLENGES
      Clogged Ducts
      Mastitis
      Breast/Chest Lymph Massage
   CHOOSING NOT TO LACTATE
   WEANING

BEYOND THE BASICS
   UNPACKING YOUR BIRTH STORY
   RECOVERY KITS

EXERCISE

CHAPTER 1

Caring for the Postpartum
Body and Mind

FUNCTION AND FEELING OVER APPEARANCE

Not long after Courtney gave birth, her husband made an offhand remark: "The dog hasn't been for a walk in a week." Totally innocent. And she burst into tears. All she had done in the week since she gave birth was nurse. That was it! Sometimes she nursed at night. Sometimes she nursed on the front porch. Sometimes she nursed on the couch. Often she fell asleep nursing. But she hadn't gone for a walk, and definitely not with the dog. The baby was too small for a front pack or stroller. Courtney had hemorrhaged after delivering the placenta and was severely anemic, and any time she walked farther than the kitchen, she started passing clots the size of eggs. But even though her whole being was telling her to just rest, she couldn't shake her guilt. So she cried. (Her husband walked the dog.)

As a twenty-five-year-old mother of one, Ruth left the hospital with a catheter in her urethra and a bag of her own urine strapped to her left leg. That night she took her jaundiced newborn, mesh panties, blood-soaked pads, saggy belly, and leaky boobs to a fiftieth birthday party. She can't remember how long she lasted. An hour? Two hours? She was exhausted. Everything hurt. She didn't know yet that she could refuse to accept invitations. She didn't like people holding her tiny human. She didn't want to take the pain pills the hospital gave her because it felt like the wrong thing to do. She was in a wilderness of the unknown with her body. She was trying to do what had served her well the rest of her life, pull up her bootstraps and get on with it. She did not rest. No one told her she should rest—or if they did tell her, she didn't listen. In her life, rest was equated with being lazy. Rest was not a sanctioned healing tool. Rest was not a natural body need. Rest was not essential. So she healed slowly, and in some cases poorly.

Bodies look and feel different postpartum than they did before pregnancy. It's normal to have strong feelings about this—maybe euphoria, delight, and amazement at the feat your body accomplished, and maybe dysphoria, unease, and dissatisfaction with your body and its mismatch with what you envision or prefer. You may feel both things at once. For many postpartum humans, pregnancy and delivery are our first major experiences with the medical system, with changes in ability, with a bodily injury that requires recovery beyond heat, ice, rest, and ibuprofen. Even excitement, love, and joy about a tiny human may be marred by a sense of *What just happened to me?*

Head-to-Toe Postpartum Body Changes

HEAD

Hormone fluctuations during and after pregnancy can impact the way you prioritize and process information. You may be more emotional than normal. Interrupted sleep patterns can leave you feeling fuzzy. The texture and amount of hair you enjoyed as a pregnant person can start to thin as your hormones shift. The muscles in your neck and shoulders may feel tense all the time.

ARMS AND SHOULDERS

Patterns of stiffness and tension in your rib and back muscles can put your arms and shoulders at a mechanical disadvantage; usually there is increased upper back rounding, made more prevalent by breastfeeding/chestfeeding. Some people develop arm weakness after months of pregnancy that causes you to use your arms less. You don't use it, you lose it! This can be harder after cesarean births when it hurts to use your core to lift, push, pull, or carry.

RIBS

Your ribs and intercostal muscles lift and stiffen in pregnancy, so your ribs may flare more or at a different angle than they used to, and the girth of your rib cage may increase. This will flatten your diaphragm, alter your breathing pattern, and can also contribute to shortness of breath.

BREAST/CHEST

The size and shape of your breasts/chest will enlarge, feeling dramatically different within the first week. Often cup size increases. The expansion of your rib cage can cause your bra band size to increase, as can weight gain. The breasts/chest are filling quickly after delivery and can be uncomfortable. Your areolas and nipples may darken and enlarge.

BACK

You overuse your back muscles to compensate for the weakness or underuse of your core, the thoracic spine stiffens, the lumbar spine sways forward.

ABDOMEN

The abdominal muscles elongate and may separate in the front. The deep core can be weak and hard to find. You may find your once full, hard belly is now sagging and wrinkled; it might have color variations (darker or lighter) and tiger stripes. Your belly may stay soft and round for a while, and people may inappropriately assume that you're still pregnant. People who have had cesarean births will be very sore, with a postoperative bandage in place, and will have a hard time with any position change for a few weeks.

PELVIC GIRDLE

The pelvic girdle expands internally and the bones flare outward; the symphysis pubis and sacroiliac joints loosen at the ligaments. The hip rotators and groin muscles may become overly mobile. Pelvic floor muscles (PFM) are pulled wider and can become hard to find. Your genitals or soft organs are going to be bleeding for several weeks. This is not going to feel like a period; it's much more swollen and tender. It may hurt to sit too long. You may have incontinence or the inability to pee after having a catheter. Your first bowel movement can take a few days to occur and feel worse than giving birth due to the inflammation of your entire pelvic region.

GLUTES AND LEGS

The hamstrings and gluteal muscles may be weaker due to shifts in your center of gravity (which keeps you upright). Your quads and hip flexor muscles may be tight and functionally weak and not able to do as much work/activity or for as long a time. You may feel like you cannot stand without leaning on something. Grocery shopping can feel like a marathon.

FEET

Your feet flatten and widen at the ligaments and tendons, causing weakness and widening of the walking pattern. Shock absorption may work less effectively, causing more strain on the back and pelvic floor. You may have swollen feet/legs for a few weeks. Your prenatal shoes may not fit.

CARDIOVASCULAR

Your heart and lungs are fundamentally altered. You may feel extremely deconditioned, as if you have never been in shape or fit in your entire life.

You may get winded, be short of breath, and need to lie down more than you ever thought was normal.

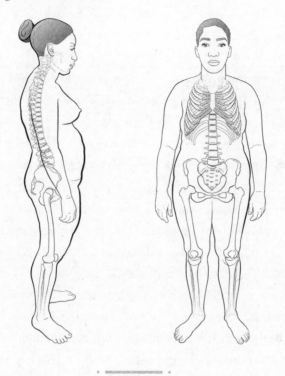

If we are not medically trained, then what we connect with is what we can see and feel. If we spent months taking pictures of our growing belly, we notice how it looks now, somewhat like a deflated balloon. The skin is not resilient yet and the abdominal muscles are also recovering, so it's holding the pregnancy shape. The uterus is going through a process called involution: shrinking and increasing in tone, too. Presentation of the belly shape, texture, and sensation will depend on how the uterus is doing in its recovery, more so if you had a cesarean birth. The pelvic floor has responded to birth and delivery with either lengthening or tensing and is often inflamed as you shed lochia or recover from vaginal/genital delivery injuries. The body and brain are tired, so tired. Our emotional hearts are living on our sleeves. Our breasts/chests are tender as we decide whether to encourage or cease lactation. Our internal organs are sluggish and have trouble doing their best work. How our body feels, looks, functions, fits in clothes, and moves may be enormously different from what we are used to. It can be hard to keep up with it all. Most of us will want all the naps.

Our postpartum healing paradigm is often distorted by the lens of the world we live in. In a supportive birth environment that fosters care, nurturing, and priority of health for the woman or birthing parent as well as the baby, you may feel tired but truly elated and may be experiencing more joy and love than you ever thought possible. This act of bringing life into the world may edify every good experience you have ever had and swell your heart. Those who are experiencing a lack of support or of a partner, poor healthcare, an infant that goes to a neonatal intensive care unit (NICU), or loss may have a difficult time. You simply may be struggling. Birth can be both beautiful and devastating.

You may also be dealing with internalized misogyny or fatphobia, or may have defined ideas about what your postpartum body "should" look like. Ruth hears this often from patients who are holding back tears. "My friend Becky just bounced right back." "Why is this happening to me?" "Why is this so hard for me?" "I am having a hard time just getting dressed in the morning." "I haven't bought new clothes yet; I keep hoping *this* [belly/boobs/ass/love handles] will go away." A sense of body betrayal can develop during your pregnancy, as both people you know and perfect strangers make comments. It might have felt okay because it wasn't a moral failing (if fatphobic) on your part; after all, you were growing a human. But the seeds are planted, waiting to sprout when we *can* do something about it. Now you have arrived, and you still look pregnant. This is absolutely the norm, but those (potentially) well-intentioned comments may be giving you ideas that you need to "do" something about your body. Sometimes these ideas override your actual need for rest, hydration, nutrition, and support. It is vital that we shift our focus to providing your body what it needs for total health, instead of idealizing its former state and lamenting how it looks now, what size pants you wear, or what that scale says. This is not the time for weight loss, dieting, or calorie counting. Buy the new clothes. Becky probably did, and just forgot to mention it. Choose what is best for you and your healing, as opposed to what you think society expects of you. When we combine body expectations with the caregiving commonly expected of the birthing parent and meeting the needs of others, a strain is placed on postpartum mental health. We need you to be mentally healthy and okay. You need it. The people in your life need it.

Hierarchy of Body Needs for Healing and Recovery

Prioritizing your recovery gives you a framework in which to navigate the dueling messages given to you by your body and societal expectations. Healing from the inside out is how you live your most vibrant life. Health in body, mind, and spirit occurs when you set healing priorities and boundaries to keep out what depletes you.

Absolute Needs During the First Six Weeks of Postpartum Recovery

1. **Rest** whenever you can get it. Ask for help from whoever is in your support network to give you resting opportunities.
2. **Hydration**, liquids that the body can use to lubricate your insides and rid you of waste. Water is best!
3. **Nutrition**, aka FOOD, for muscle healing, scar healing, possibly milk production, and energy. Feed yourself accordingly.
4. **Support** by saying no to things that interfere with your needs and saying yes to things and people that make you feel nourished.

If you find that you are not giving yourself the care you need—not eating, resting, or socializing—seek out mental health services or a trusted medical professional. Outside voices can do an efficient job of eroding our self-esteem, particularly if we have learned to place our value as humans on what we look like and how we can be of service to others, and are now juggling a new role like being a parent. Sometimes it's our inner critic that is hurting our recovery by not prioritizing healing. It's worth the time and energy to learn how to nurture and love yourself now, and every day. Mental health issues occur in one in five postpartum humans and are the leading cause of death in the fourth trimester. Ask for the support you need so you can recover and thrive—we'll cover this topic in greater depth in chapter 3.

The purpose of rest and care is to support your body in fulfilling its myriad roles and responsibilities. In addition to the typical sleeping/thinking/metabolizing/interacting functions you perform all the time, your postpartum body is also engaged in the healing of tissues and organs and hormonal signaling for sleep, hunger, stress, fluid management, and mood. If you're caring for a newborn, you're adding feeding (possibly including milk production), diaper changing, holding, rocking, bouncing, and so on. Not to mention maintaining your home, and maybe working. All these activities take a toll similar to a highway toll, in that you have to pay for them. They accept the currencies of rest, hydration, nutrition, and social support. The more your body and mind do, the more you must pay. When there's an imbalance between performance and cost, you open the door to physical or mental dysfunction.

How do you know if you are giving yourself the kind of care your body needs? Watch for indications that you are depleting or overstraining your system. The feelings and sensations in your body are like a report card on the balance of activity versus currency. Some common aches and pains are:

- Heaviness in your belly and pelvic floor
- Leaking urine or increased bleeding with activity
- Back and pelvic pain

10

- Headaches
- Intractable fatigue
- Gastrointestinal (GI) upset

Listen to and respect your body's communication. Ignoring its signals can lead to injury, body shame, mood dysregulation, burnout, and postpartum depression. This is a plea to push back against leaning into more. Don't lean in, lean out. If you are having any of the above symptoms, ask yourself how you can lighten the load. How can you give your body ease?

The basic needs of the postpartum human are rest, hydration, nutrition, and support on your terms.

REST

Rest is the cornerstone of healing. Rest is recovery. Rest is essential. Rest is a natural body need. Rest is an evidence-based healing tool. Rest and recovery fuel your nervous system. Rest allows your brain to function— after all, "mom brain" is just a symptom of exhaustion. Rest supports compassionate thought, mental health, arousal and sexual interest, and pooping. Not all rest is sleep, but you need that, too—six hours minimum in a twenty-four-hour period. Up to ten would have you feeling much better, but for many postpartum humans this isn't entirely up to you. Again, ask for help from family, friends, neighbors, or your partner to do the things that keep you from sleeping. Ask for a meal train. Say no to guests who want you to make them a snack. Say yes to guests who *bring* you a snack. Explore your own bandwidth. If you don't want guests staying in your house, but your extended family can't live another second without holding your tiny human, tell them to get a room nearby. Be explicit regarding how long a visit is helpful rather than harmful to your healing.

Rest is easier said than done. American society isn't built for you. There's no federally mandated paid parental leave policy, and state laws vary wildly, from no protections to some paid leave. You might need to return to work as soon as two weeks after delivery, for job security and to pay the bills. This is before you've stopped shedding lochia, before you've been cleared to exercise, before your six-week checkup. For those privileged enough to have any leave time, you might still feel the pressure to exercise or even return to work earlier than is required.

Then there's the fact that life doesn't stop just because you grew a human. You might have other children, pets, or elder dependents. You might look upon the mess of dishes, laundry, toys, books, whatever, and despair. Many of us are not good at asking for help and view ourselves as strong, independent people—we *want* to be someone who can do it all. We're conditioned to think we can just work a little harder and make it all happen. All of us have experienced the shame and letdown that occurs when we end the day with items left undone on our to-do list. Essentially, "getting things done" is a shame spiral. If you are a to-do list person, put *nap* at the top of the list every day. Go ahead and add *heal* as well. It's happening in the background whether you recognize it or not, so you might as well give yourself credit.

We're not saying those asks are easy, but we are giving you permission. Your body and your healing must stay on the priority list, and sadly that hasn't yet been normalized. So consider your needs. What will allow you to rest and let your body do what it needs to do to both heal and take care of the new human? How can you resist the nagging feeling that you should be doing more?

For those of you who have always been type A and need to see the stats, more smart watches are now tracking stress level, sleep, heart rate, and heart rate variability. Seeing the hard data about our lack of REM and deep sleep, or about the prolonged period of time it takes for our heart rate to drop at night, can be a catalyst to give ourselves what we need. Look into devices that track these things and compare your vital statistics now to your pregnant and prenatal self. This can be a tangible way to determine your stress versus rest cycles during the day, and to differentiate the people who allow you to access your resting self from those who stress you out and further deplete your battery. You might prefer to keep track of your stress and rest in a journal, documenting your subjective experience and noticing patterns.

If tracking is too cumbersome or feels triggering, use your intuition. Which types of activities let you settle into rest? How does your body feel when you are around certain people? Do you feel calm, open, relaxed, and grounded? Or do you feel tense, strained, hypervigilant, and anxious? Choose activities and people who soothe you.

HYDRATION

Hydration refers both to the fluid you drink and the ability of your body systems to use that fluid. Hydration is often misunderstood, and there aren't many well-designed research studies concerning postpartum needs for hydration. As always, your body is your best ally. This doesn't mean just "drink when you're thirsty." That means paying attention. When you are adequately hydrated, your body can process everything more efficiently. Drinking *enough* prevents muscle cramps, headaches, nausea, bladder irritation, constipation, and fatigue. There is research to indicate that drinking enough water feeds your brain, making you more relaxed, with improved cognitive function, attention, memory, and mood. Now, who doesn't need that?

So how much water is enough? The Institute of Medicine and the National Academy of Sciences recommend 77–91 ounces per day for nineteen- to fifty-year-old women or those assigned female at birth. However, that number takes into consideration water you get from food, which is hard to measure, but is estimated at 25 percent of your daily intake. So aim for 48–64 fluid ounces of water per day, and more if you're losing water through sweat.

Here's the but. Anything to do with numbers can trigger obsessive thoughts, as if there is a right/wrong decision to be made. Some of us obsess that more is always better. Numbers don't tell you anything about how to *feel*, so throw them out if they don't work for you. As it stands, there is no standard estimated average requirement, because the requirements are based on a combination of health factors, like body size, activity level, external environment, and chronic health conditions. Those who are pregnant or lactating have an estimated higher need. Your ability to listen to your body and intuition are your most important tools.

Barriers to hydration may be limiting your water intake—out of sight, out of mind. If you're couch- or bed-bound (own your rest!), keeping a large water bottle nearby takes away one of those barriers. Many of our interviewees told us about their favorite water bottles, including the hospital-grade jug with a straw. If your public drinking water quality is poor, this is a place you can ask for deliveries of water from your support system. Just bad at drinking? Ruth uses the water bottle technique to train her clients who are drinking less than 48 ounces to meet the minimum. Figure out how much you need to drink each day and fill containers with that amount. Put them somewhere as a visual reminder. Use more than one bottle if you move from room to room a lot or are always looking for your water. Set short-term goals like "by lunch I will drink two bottles," and sip throughout the day.

Besides bladder irritation and slow bowels, the earliest signs of dehydration include thirst, dry mouth, darker urine, fatigue, and flushed skin. This is the time to increase your water intake. If you do not and develop symptoms that the dehydration is getting worse—increased body temperature, heart rate, or rate of breathing; diarrhea; fever; vomiting; or heat exhaustion—you need to go to the emergency department.

Overhydrating is possible, too. Ruth has clients with a well-intentioned daily intake of water at some percentage of their body weight. Let's be honest: this practice is often rooted in diet culture—what diet program isn't peddling water consumption to cut down caloric intake and hunger? But water intake alone does not give you the nutrients you need to heal. Food is not the bad guy. In fact, research suggests that protein intake with water intake improves overall hydration and muscle recovery after sport. You were pregnant and now you are healing (and likely taking on a demanding role called parenting), which we consider an endurance sport. Don't use water as a meal replacement or a way to reduce hunger.

There are no clear recommendations on maximum water intake per day. As a precaution, a limit of 128 ounces, which is a gallon, is suggested. Symptoms you might be hydrating too much include frequent or excessive urination, never feeling empty after urinating, bladder pain, incontinence, nighttime urination, and urine that is always clear. Other body symptoms include headaches, nausea, unsteady or weak muscles, exhaustion, disorientation, swollen feet/hands/lips, and low blood sugar. A rare but serious condition called hyponatremia can occur when you drink so much water that it causes low sodium in your body, which can be life-threatening and requires emergency medical care. Symptoms of hyponatremia include dizziness, fatigue, nausea, vomiting, cramping, headache, and sleepiness.

Listen to your body needs, watch your urine, and monitor symptoms to determine what is right for you. Remember that your body needs electrolytes to be balanced for heart and tissue happiness, and too much water depletes that. Please fight the idea that more is always better or there is only one way to do things.

Not all liquids are equally hydrating, and some can exacerbate bladder dysfunction. Bladder irritants can increase our urine production, fill our bladder faster, irritate our bladder lining, or mess with the relationship between the nervous system and pelvic floor health, altering our organ's emptying cues and ability to fully empty. This could be particularly uncomfortable while your pelvic floor is healing.

Bladder irritants include:

- Coffee (even decaf)
- Black, green, oolong, and chai teas

- Chocolate (to drink or to eat)
- Carbonated beverages (including seltzer, soda, kombucha, and kefir)
- Artificial sweeteners like aspartame or sucralose
- Nicotine
- Alcohol

An irritated organ can be painful and empty more frequently or with more urgency. This can lead to incontinence and/or retention. Neither is pleasant. We recommend that at least 50 percent of your fluid intake be water, starting on the lower end if you're accustomed to drinking other beverages and building up to 48 ounces per day. If you're experiencing bladder or bowel irritation and aren't sure what could be the cause, you can try eliminating one potential irritant at a time, for a few days at a time. Then add it back in and notice any improvements in your bowel or bladder function and feeling. You can also try eliminating all potential irritants at once for four days to two weeks. You'll learn a lot about your body, and you'll be able to make informed choices. If you love coffee, and you find that it is an irritant, you still get to make the choice as to whether you continue to drink it or not, with full knowledge of the risks and benefits. Remember, life is about balance, and that's what we are encouraging you to discover: what is right for you.

NUTRITION

Listen—giving birth is the Uterus Olympics. Your body completed ten months of intense preparation for one pinnacle performance. Elite and professional athletes have a behind-the-scenes team preparing their specially crafted meals, tailored to their needs. Olympian Michael Phelps reportedly consumed 8,000 to 10,000 calories per day during training and meets leading up to the Beijing Olympics, where he won eight gold medals and broke seven world records. You brought one human into this world, and you got a hospital tray. You deserve the right amounts and types of fuel for your amazing feats, too. Too often we view food as our enemy, basing our self-worth on what we consume and paying too close attention to numbers that are not easily calculated, like calories. Shift your mindset to see food as fuel to feed your healing and your ability to live the life you want. A deprived body is not a body that feels good. Your body is your home. Fuel it like you are an impeccable athlete who just completed the Uterus Olympics and who is now beginning a new event, the Postpartum Period.

The word *diet* literally means what you eat. Figuratively, diet refers to a caloric or nutrient deficit used to induce weight loss. This is not the time to start a weight-loss diet. This is the time to focus on giving your body nutrition. Calories are a way that energy in food is measured. We need energy in our diet, but a calorie count can be misleading. It doesn't tell you what the body needs or the total nutrition you are getting; it's telling you the immediate available energy of that food. From now on, let's ditch the word *diet* and refer to food based on its nutritional value.

Fiber and protein are the two nutritional staples that will help you heal and are worth paying attention to the numbers on. Aim for 28 to 35 grams of fiber per day. On your standard nutrition facts label, fiber is listed under carbohydrates and is found in whole foods like fruits, vegetables, legumes, nuts, seeds, and grains. Aim to "eat the rainbow" (not Skittles, sorry) and get fiber from a variety of foods.

Recommended amounts of protein vary, but you should aim for 46 grams per day if you aren't lactating and 71 per day if you are. Another recent recommendation is 1.7 grams of protein for every kilogram of body weight. In the nonmetric system, that would be 125 grams of protein per day for a person who weighs 165 pounds. The type of protein you eat will also have a bearing on the type and quantity of fat you consume. Meat-based and plant-based proteins have different nutritional profiles, and you get to choose, based on your preferences and how your body feels best. Courtney is a vegetarian, and Ruth brought her fiber- and protein-rich falafel while in the hospital. For those who are vegetarian or vegan, there are special recommendations for you. Speak to your doctor about how to supplement micronutrients you may not be getting, like vitamin B_{12}, iron, calcium, and zinc.

Food is also a bridge to our communities. It is a way we connect with people around us. Sharing a meal promotes togetherness and comfort. Someone cooking our favorite dish is an act of love. Your cultural community might have dishes or ingredients specific to the postpartum period. If your favorite or culturally significant foods don't fall into a category of nutritional "perfection," it's okay. You are allowed to enjoy food for its own sake. It doesn't have to serve a particular function. Sometimes it's okay to feed your heart and mind in the service of connection to your loved ones and your community.

Your overall nutrition will affect a significant aspect of your well-being: poop. As Ruth tells her patients, if you want to be regular, you have to be regular! The bowel moves consistently when it is filling consistently. We have an urge to empty about 20 minutes after eating each meal, and regular folks tend to empty at the same time every day. Fiber will hold the stool together and will help us empty more completely. You may experience constipation in the first week or two. Before adding a lot of fiber that could be too filling and cause too large a bowel movement, try increasing your fluid intake. Don't take a fiber supplement for this same reason—a large movement is hard to pass. Stool softeners can take the edge off and make emptying less painful. Get your knees higher than your hips, using a stool or a Squatty Potty. Do *not* force that poop out. Breathe to relax your pelvic floor. Hum on the toilet or make raspberry or horse lips sounds instead of straining. This protects your pelvic organs and your pelvic floor from injury.

Bowel movements can be a sign about how you are doing with the big three—rest, hydration, and nutrition—because they are regulated by our parasympathetic nervous system. Some people call this the "rest and digest" nervous system. If we are regulating ourselves and recovering well from childbirth and delivery, and we are hydrating and eating well, then our bowels will regulate themselves.

It's all well and good for us to make these recommendations, but we know that eating well can be difficult in general, much less during the paradigm shift associated with being postpartum. Here are a few things you can try to make mealtime less stressful:

- Buying precut and washed fruits and vegetables or asking others to bring them to you.

- Buying canned or frozen fruits, legumes, and vegetables to reduce food waste and make preparation easier.

- Combining protein and fiber in the form of shakes, smoothies, and soups.

- Get on that meal train! When people ask what they can do to help, be specific. Have someone coordinate food deliveries/drop-offs from your loved ones.

- Ask people to buy you something during their own grocery shopping that they can deliver to your door. In those first few weeks, it can be daunting just to grab a bottle of milk or toilet paper. This is especially necessary for those in a food desert or with transportation issues.

Every person we interviewed stated they loved and valued their meal train or wished they'd had one. Who knew feeding yourself could be so fraught? Ask for help, be specific about what you need, and cut yourself slack if the outcome is not what you imagined the ideal to be.

Here's one simple and delicious way to get the protein and fiber that will nourish and strengthen you.

SYLVIA'S BLACK BEANS

When Courtney was three weeks postpartum, her in-laws came to visit. She was anemic during this time, and the baby began cluster feeding as soon as company arrived. Her mother-in-law, Sylvia, who is Guatemalan, immediately made a huge pot of black beans. She started with two cups of dry beans and cooked them for about four hours over low heat in eight cups of water, with half of an onion cut in two pieces, three whole garlic cloves, and two teaspoons of salt. The beans were delicious, but what really made Courtney happy was the mugful of the cooking liquid that Sylvia handed her that afternoon. It was warm, savory, and iron-rich, and as she sipped it, she felt better than she had in a long time. Serve the beans with the liquid as soup, adding chopped-up vegetables or meat for more variety. You can also strain the beans, sauté them with a little olive oil and chopped onion, and eat them with rice, enjoy with toppings like avocado or jalapeño peppers, or use them to fill tacos or burritos with eggs—whatever is easy and sounds delicious. You can use canned black beans as well, for even greater ease, but the cooking liquid won't be quite as magical.

SUPPORT

None of us is built to do this parenting thing alone, heal alone, or recover from grief or trauma alone. They are highly social experiences that depend on robust support systems to help us in ways we cannot always intellectualize and demarcate. Gathering your friends, family, and social networks in a supportive community is an essential piece of the puzzle. These folks may help you with meals and meal planning to support your nutritional needs. They may offer emotional support and social experiences that rebuild, rather than deplete, your energy. They can complete some of your tasks on that endless to-do list to give you opportunities to rest, sleep, and use your body's energy for healing. They can offer you playfulness and joy. They will treat you like a whole person, not just your pregnancy/postpartum identity—and converse about anything you like, from current events to good books.

Your community will also respect your need for space: time to reconcile with your new identity, to bond with your new human, and to reshape your relationship with your family. Invite them in when their presence nourishes you, and don't when it won't. You don't owe anyone outside of your immediate family your time and energy right now.

THE ROLE OF HORMONES IN POSTPARTUM RECOVERY

During pregnancy, your hormones underwent drastic shifts, and they continue to evolve. The progesterone, estrogen, and relaxin that surged during pregnancy drop immediately after. Prolactin and oxytocin rush in, anticipating lactation and bonding. When they taper off, around six weeks postpartum, symptoms of postpartum depression and/or anxiety may emerge.

Symptoms of hormonal imbalance include mood swings, low libido, vaginal/genital dryness, abdominal pain related to ovarian or uterine conditions, unexpected weight fluctuations, or even more profound exhaustion, so it's worth mentioning any of these to your provider. Postpartum thyroiditis, a condition in which the thyroid becomes inflamed after pregnancy, occurs in about 5 percent of people. Symptoms depend on whether the thyroid is over- or underactive, but can include anxiety, an increased heart rate, warmth, unexpected weight loss, and muscle weakness (overactive), or coldness, fatigue, constipation, brain fog, and unexpected weight gain (underactive). These symptoms could also indicate another hormone-related condition, so letting your provider know when you notice any of them will hopefully get you appropriate care. Enlist your advocates if needed!

If you used to take any sort of hormone therapy—say, for birth control or relief of period symptoms—or hormone replacement therapy (HRT) for gender affirmation, you likely stopped while pregnant. When to resume treatments depends on several factors. Generally, you may resume hormonal birth control after your six-week checkup. If you're feeding through lactation, you may be prescribed a low-dose pill or have an IUD inserted instead. There is a fairly standard set of recommendations here.

However, there aren't any standard recommendations for when to resume HRT postpartum. According to trans gestational parent and educator Trystan Reese, anyone planning to do so should do a "cost-benefit analysis" of what will best support their mental and physical health. He chose to postpone HRT until he felt physically on the upswing following a hemorrhage during delivery and used topical estradiol to assist with wet tissue healing. Reese also knows trans gestational parents who resumed HRT while still in the hospital. It's about what will affirm you and help you heal in whatever way you need. The mental health and identity aspects of postpartum recovery may be much more important to your overall wellness than the secondary benefits of estrogen and postpartum hormonal changes. You can choose to have a plan in place ahead of birth or wait and see what feels best based on your healing.

LACTATION AND CESSATION OF LACTATION

We will be using the word lactation *throughout this section to describe the production of milk from your body. We will be using the words* breastfeeding/chestfeeding *to describe a tiny human drinking milk directly from the body. Pumping and expressing milk are also ways milk can be removed from the body and fed to a tiny human.*

Breast Milk/Human Milk: What Is It?

Your body has been producing a milklike substance since week 14 to 16 of pregnancy. This will account for the heaviness you feel in your breasts/chest with each passing week. You may have even leaked in the weeks leading up to delivery or intentionally expressed some to bank it for later. This beginning "milk" is called colostrum.

Colostrum is a thick yellowish secretion containing nutrients and other immune-enhancing bioactive components. Its color and nutrient density are what give it the nickname "liquid gold." These nutritive substances offer protection to the tiny human, especially as they have never eaten by mouth before. Colostrum coats an infant's intestines, protecting from infection and acting as a laxative. This is especially important for clearing out meconium, the first infant poop, from their digestive system.

Because all pregnant humans develop colostrum from week 14 to 16 of pregnancy, all deliveries after this time will result in colostrum in the breasts. After delivery, whether you encourage lactation through nursing or pumping will determine if transitional, and then mature, milk comes in.

Encouraging Lactation

Skip ahead to Choosing Not to Lactate (page 32) if you are not planning to encourage lactation!
After the first three days of feeding or pumping, you will develop transitional milk. This milk is whiter than colostrum and has more calories. You will notice breast/chest engorgement, tightening skin around the breasts/chest and areolas, leaking, and increased supply. This can be delayed due to poor latch, infrequent feeding or pumping, hormone imbalances, anemia, high blood pressure, and other chronic health conditions.

Mature milk will come in between ten and fourteen days postpartum. It is thin and white and resembles skim milk. Its fat content changes during a feed, becoming fattier and more nutrient dense at the end. That's why it is important to feed entirely from one side before switching to the other, especially for babies struggling to gain weight.

Lactation:
An Issue of Rights and Privilege

Lactation offers some measurable benefits to you. It can reduce your risk of certain cancers, cardiovascular and hypertensive diseases, and type 2 diabetes. It can increase your production of oxytocin, a hormone that helps with mood, bonding with your baby, and your uterus returning to size following delivery. You may have been inundated with these and similar factoids as reasons that you *must* breastfeed/chestfeed, but what these well-intentioned facts dismiss is the human cost of lactation.

In our society, lactation is a privilege. It is not a "free" method. It takes time and space, whether you are expressing milk via a pump or feeding the baby directly. It requires a lot of energy and can be exhausting, as it may put most of the feeding responsibility on you, the birthing parent. Having the support to sleep in after a hard night's feeding, being at home during the day to lactate on demand, or having the supplies, equipment, and time to pump at your workplace to maintain your supply could be the determining factors of your lactation success.

Medical, economic, social, and workplace circumstances often play heavily into how feasible it is to use lactation to feed a baby. Due to systemic inequities present in the United States, breastfeeding/chestfeeding may be more or less accessible to you. It also means that if you plan to feed through lactation and find that it isn't possible, you aren't alone. Nationally, 83.9 percent of birthing parents breastfeed/chestfeed sometimes, with 56.7 percent continuing at six months, and 35 percent after a year. We can't recommend breastfeeding/chestfeeding over other forms of feeding until we have universal paid parental leave, equitable enactment of existing pumping laws, free supplies for pumping, and reduced stigma about feeding method.

Supports for Lactation Success

If you are planning to feed through lactation, here are some resources and tips to support your success.

EDUCATION AND BIRTHING FACILITY RESOURCES

Know what lactation support and education is available in your birthing facility. Ideally, you will have access to lactation consultants during your stay, and you will know how to contact them with questions after you're discharged. The Affordable Care Act mandates coverage for up to six lactation consultations, which can start before delivery. Lactation consultants can guide you in getting your milk to come in, helping your baby to latch, and feeling comfortable while breastfeeding/chestfeeding. They can also help with weaning and working on never having your milk come in, if that is your choice.

Know your facility's policies regarding having the baby in your room all day, also known as 24-hour rooming-in, and if they promote and allow early skin-to-skin contact, regardless of birthing method. The World Health Association correlates 90 minutes of skin-to-skin contact immediately after birth with a 90 percent success rate in feeding through lactation.

Lactation consultant Paula Norcott, IBCLC, recommends effective stimulation or milk removal eight to ten times a day with baby or a quality pump, or hand expression, to encourage the development of a full milk supply. Finding the balance between sleep and a milk removal schedule with no breaks longer than four hours is a challenge, but evidence suggests that eight milk removal sessions each day for the first four weeks can go a long way in establishing your supply.

WORKPLACE PROVISIONS FOR PUMPING

If you're planning to work while feeding through lactation, find out what provisions your workplace offers. Federal law requires employers to provide reasonable break time for an employee to express milk for their child for one year after the child's birth each time such employee has a need to express the milk (Section 7 of the Fair Labor Standards Act). Employers are also required to provide a place, other than a bathroom, that is shielded from view and free from intrusion from coworkers and the public, which may be used by an employee to express milk. However, what this looks like and how strictly it's adhered to are (unfortunately) highly variable.

Not all pumps are created equal. See what is covered through your insurance and start there. Hands-free models have improved a lot, and there are some that can fit entirely within a nursing bra with no hoses or tubes hanging out. If your goal is to multitask while pumping, these can be beneficial. It's also okay to use expressing milk as an opportunity to take a break and rest. In fact, some people get a better milk supply when they use their pumping time to relax and focus on letdown, rather than being busy with other tasks.

ACCESSORIES

Whether you're pumping or feeding directly, lactation can be uncomfortable. For some people, their nipples crack, milk leaks, and feeding in public feels awkward and embarrassing. Here are a few products which we—and the people we interviewed—recommend, which will hopefully make life easier as you transition into a more comfortable relationship with lactation/feeding:

* Safe-to-ingest nipple creams, with coconut, olive oil, or lanolin bases

- Easy-access tops and bras
- Pads to absorb leaking milk
- Nipple or nursing shields, if recommended by a professional for a more effective latch
- Milk freezer storage bags if you're expressing milk for later use

Breastfeeding/Chestfeeding Basics

Given that one of our defining characteristics as mammals is the fact that we can produce milk to feed our young, it's surprising how difficult it can be to get the hang of it. Here's a rundown of the basics.

Holding your baby so that you're comfortable and they can easily latch and suckle prompts your body to release oxytocin, signaling your body to let down milk, and prolactin, signaling your body to produce milk. (The action of a pump aims to trigger the same hormonal response.) Try sitting, lying on your side, and holding the baby in various safe positions to see what works for you. Pillows, including donut-like nursing pillows with cute covers, can be strategically placed to support your back and arms.

How your baby latches and how well they suckle milk will determine how well they are fed. If you're concerned that they aren't latching or suckling effectively—perhaps they aren't gaining weight or seem excessively hungry or fussy; you're not feeling emptied after feeding or are becoming engorged; or your nipples are cracked, bruised, or otherwise painful—check in with a lactation consultant, pediatrician, your healthcare provider, or another resource. Sometimes these things can be remedied with an adjustment in positioning, but they can be indicative of a lip- or tongue-tie or other anatomical difference. For Courtney, lactation and feeding were challenging in the first week. Her milk production occurred later than expected due to her postpartum anemia, and her baby had a tongue-tie, which was observed and rectified by her pediatrician within a few days of delivery. Due to concerns around her baby's weight gain, they supplemented with formula for a little while and then proceeded with breast milk as a primary food source.

If your schedule allows, feeding based on the baby's hunger signals—that is to say, feeding until the baby shows signs of being full (i.e., pops off the nipple)—allows your milk supply to keep up with demand. Many folks can achieve feeding on demand only if all they are doing is caring for their baby. If feeding on a schedule is what works best for you both, then do that.

Lactation Challenges

It's common to experience engorgement, or tenderness and pain due to fullness, in the first three to five days after delivery. It can be a chaotic 72 hours of establishing your milk supply. Engorgement occurs in 50 to 75 percent of newly lactating parents, but it doesn't have to happen; according to Norcott, the underlying cause is inflammation, not the status of your milk supply. Treat inflammation with ice and anti-inflammatory medication such as ibuprofen to reduce any discomfort, or place cabbage leaves (yes, really) against the inflamed tissue, which release a soothing chemical while they wilt. You can also try hand-expressing milk and breastfeeding or pumping every three hours or as needed to reduce swelling and improve your comfort. Avoid overfeeding or extra pumping, as that puts you into a supply-and-demand cycle that *increases* production.

CLOGGED DUCTS
Clogged ducts can be caused by overproduction of milk, too much pressure from a bra, and a lack of our big three (rest, hydration, and nutrition). This presents as a small, painful, slightly swollen area on one side, with a bruise-like sensation. A plug can often be dislodged through breastfeeding, hand-expressing, or pumping. Using a Haakaa pump with Epsom

salts is another popular way to clear a clogged milk duct, or you can try gentle lymphatic massage. Some doctors and lactation consultants recommend taking lecithin to prevent recurring blockages, but no clinical studies have validated if it is safe or effective for this purpose. Let your physician know about any blockages that don't resolve within a few days, or increased swelling, pain, or a fever.

MASTITIS

Mastitis, the big bad of lactation woes, is caused by a staph infection in the breast/top tissue and remains rare. Common causes include stasis of the milk supply (not enough emptying sessions), nipple breakdown and cracking, introduction of bacteria through these cracks via your tiny human's mouth, and high stress levels. If you spot pus or yellow discharge, have it tested in a lab for bacteria as soon as possible to catch an infection before it gets any worse. Symptoms of mastitis include pain, tenderness, inflammation, fever, flu-like chills and achiness, and systemic illness that becomes worse over time. It is no joke. Get medical attention immediately and take whatever antibiotics they give you. If the antibiotics don't work on the first round, seek further treatment.

Courtney got acute onset mastitis after ten months of breastfeeding, and it wasn't pretty: nausea, vomiting, a fever of 103 degrees, blacking out, two rounds of antibiotics, and days completely out of commission. It's crucial to continue breastfeeding/chestfeeding or pumping during mastitis to prevent worsening infection and further stasis of milk in the breast/top tissue.

BREAST/CHEST LYMPH MASSAGE

Lymphatic massage is a *very* gentle stroking of the breast/top tissue with the tips of your fingers. Avoid using a lot of pressure, no more than the weight of nickel, to reduce the risk of compressing the milk ducts or increasing tissue inflammation that could lead to more pain and problems. This is not therapeutic massage or trying to "bust the clog." The purpose is reducing the swelling in your breast/top tissue to allow a clog, swelling, or milk stasis to resolve. You can do this dry with gentle fingers or with massage oil or coconut oil. Choose something without a fragrance.

1. Sit or lie somewhere comfortable. Put the arm on the same side as the involved breast/top tissue over your head. Gently stroke from underneath the armpit upward to just above shoulder level in a sweeping motion. This is where most of your lymph nodes reside and ensures that you are not pushing fluid into an already "full" area. Perform 3 to 5 strokes.

2. Sweep from sternum to armpit, like following the tip of a butterfly's wing, over the top of the breast/top tissue and underneath the lower third of the breast/top tissue. Perform 3 to 5 strokes.

3. Make gentle fingertip circles with your index, middle, and ring finger around the areola. Do 3 circles in one small space; then move one inch to the side and repeat. Your other hand may cup the heavier part of the breast/top tissue to make this more comfortable. Do this clockwise and counterclockwise.

4. Cup your hands around the large part of the breast/top tissue, positioning your hands thumb to thumb and fingertips to fingertips. Perform a gentle sweep from the large part of the tissue to the areola. Repeat 3 to 5 strokes.

5. From the larger part of the breast/top tissue to the areola, perform contrasting sweeps with each hand, one pulling to the chest and one pulling to the areola. Repeat around the entire area.

6. Use your fingers to cup the underside of the breast/top tissue and pull the fingers away from one another. Sweep up and around to the top. Repeat 3 to 5 strokes.

7. Repeat the first step 3 to 5 times for a final evacuation of the fluid to the lymph nodes in the armpit. Follow up with ice, the Haakaa, or feeding to continue to promote lactation and reduce the risk of further stasis in the ducts.

Lactation does not come easily to everyone. There are a lot of factors that play into why it might not be working for you or your baby. If you are feeling overwhelmed or resentful, or you dread your time feeding or pumping, please know that you don't have to continue. Some people, particularly those who are prone to depression and/or anxiety, also experience dysphoric milk ejection reflex (DMER), which can feel like anger or rage during letdown. Because lactation is a hormonally mitigated process, people respond to it in different ways. Talk to a provider if you are experiencing these feelings. They are not uncommon.

For those with prior trauma or assault experiences, having your tiny human latching to your body can feel like an invasion. Some people feel triggered by the sensations on their skin, even if they have been to therapy and are working through feelings of safety. A nipple shield can be a great resource to add a barrier of protection for your body and reduce the early negative side effects of latching, such as cracked nipples and soreness. If you want to breastfeed and are experiencing a "too much" sensation, the nipple shield can help you feed with less discomfort. You do not need to pump or feed longer with a nipple shield.

No one gets awards for lactation. A healthy postpartum human and a healthy tiny human are the goals. If you want to keep trying, seek out professionals like a lactation consultant, postpartum doula, or midwife.

If you're ready to stop, then stop.

We want *you* to be healthy in body and mind. Do what is right for you to achieve this goal.

Choosing Not to Lactate

Should you wish to prevent breast milk/human milk production alto-gether, it is important to avoid nipple stimulation while you're still pro-ducing colostrum. Binding tightly with an Ace wrap can stop it from coming in. Expressing by hand is not recommended, as that can stimulate milk production, but you can consider it in small amounts if you find your breasts are hard and full for more than 48 hours. Work with your medical provider to see if medications to stop prolactin and milk production are an option. Norcott says to expect "72 crazy hours" of icing, not removing any milk, and avoiding contact with hot water, after which milk produc-tion will decrease and then stop. She also recommends peppermint in any form—breath mints, tea, etc.—and Sudafed for drying up supply.

If you're raising a baby and know that feeding through lactation isn't for you, you may find that birthing professionals are putting pressure on you to do it regardless. This is likely due to the influences of their advisory boards, hospital and healthcare center credentialing requirements, na-tionwide lactation advocacy efforts, and their personal opinions. Let your birthing staff and healthcare center know your choice in advance. They still may be required to offer information regarding lactation benefits be-fore they can document that you are choosing not to. Have someone show you that it is documented in your medical record.

Some hospitals and birthing centers are labeled "baby-friendly." This designation can mean that they place an even greater emphasis on lacta-tion. If you have the option to choose your hospital or birthing center, you can take this into consideration. However, even a "baby-friendly" facility must listen to and honor your decisions. Norcott recommends discussing your intention not to lactate with your provider ahead of time and having that information included in your chart.

Weaning

The best solution for your comfort and to reduce the side effects of weaning is the planned, slow approach. Drop one pump or one feed per day every three days. You may also decrease pumping time by 3 to 5 minutes each session. If you have symptoms of swelling, use ice and gentle hand expression to relieve symptoms, but not too much milk. This will allow your body to adjust the supply and eventually (after about two months) stop producing milk.

Circumstances may dictate that you wean suddenly. This can cause you to have more acute symptoms, like breast/chest swelling and tenderness. Some medications can help your body stop producing milk, but that recommendation should come directly from a consultant or provider.

No matter how quickly you wean, you may experience temporary tenderness or fullness, which can be relieved by icing your breasts/chest as often as possible and/or the old favorite, cabbage leaves that you allow to wilt against your breasts/chest in a bra or other supportive garment. Perform lymphatic massage and remove milk with hand expression or a tool like the Haakaa only for comfort. If you feel more acute pain, hardness, or heat in your breasts/chest, let your healthcare provider know.

There are often big feelings associated with the decision to wean, partly because of the hormonal changes associated with weaning, but also because of the expectations society places on breastfeeding/chestfeeding and because of the emotions that come with change and the tiny human growing up. It may also come as a welcome relief. All those feelings are real and valid. Everyone's experience will be different. Observe and acknowledge how you are feeling, mentally and physically, and ask for the help you need.

Be aware, however, that a decrease in oxytocin and prolactin, and the resultant increase in estrogen, can have a significant impact on your mental health, mood, and hormone balance. You may feel like you have the baby blues again. People with a history of mood dysregulation and concerns about their mental health may want to contact their medical providers about their plans to wean and medicate proactively. If you notice changes in your typical anxiety, stress levels, or mood during or soon after weaning, let a provider in your birthing community or your primary care physician know right away, and work toward getting support through this transition.

Contrasts in Weaning

After eleven months of feeding through a combination of breastfeeding and pumping, Ruth and her tiny human realized they were ready to be done. She had made it almost to the twelve-month finish line (we did mention she's type A-minus, right?) for breastfeeding benefits. Her baby was easily distracted during feedings and was craving more independence in eating. She was able to transition to formula and solids with a steady decrease in pumping and limited offerings of nursing times. One day, they just weren't breastfeeding anymore.

In contrast, Courtney, who was ready to be done after seventeen months, found she was unable to gradually taper over the summer, when she and her toddler were together all day. When a work trip—and a distractible kid—gave her the extra nudge to stop, her body just kept on producing milk. She was painfully swollen and worried about a second case of mastitis. Additionally, the changes in hormones led to a serious decline in her mental health, including body dysmorphia. After a miserable week, she called the lactation consultant she had worked with in the hospital, who guided her to antihistamines and birth control, and eventual relief.

BEYOND THE BASICS

Unpacking Your Birth Story

What is the difference between a traumatic birth and a "normal" birth? Your perception and how you feel about what happened to you. That's it. Often, birthing people who define their experience as traumatic might not be classified as having experienced trauma by a qualified medical professional reviewing their chart. That's because there are factors that play into your feelings that can't be quantified, like how your expectations compared to the outcomes, whether you felt heard and included in the decisions made during the birth process or aftercare, feeling guilt over the birth, being overwhelmed by the experience, or knowing that what a birthing team considers normal may sound terrifying.

Here are some prompts to help you determine if you feel like you had a traumatic birth story:

* Poor birth plan compliance
* Lack of explanation of techniques used in delivery and clinical reasoning
* Lack of autonomy in birthing decisions
* Lack of respect shown by birthing staff
* Feeling lied to when offered decision-making that wasn't really possible
* Experiencing stitching without anesthesia taking full effect
* Lack of medical intervention for incontinence postpartum
* Lack of medical intervention for painful intercourse postpartum
* Lack of skin-to-skin contact with infant, interrupting bonding
* Lack of lactation support
* Partner/support person not allowed in delivery room

- Experiencing obstetric trauma: painful and numerous pelvic examinations without being told the reason or your comfort being taken seriously
- Emotional expressions of birth including powerlessness, depression, violation, fear

A medical professional can screen you for perinatal post-traumatic stress disorder (PTSD). This occurs in some 9 percent of all births and is much more likely if you had a premature birth, stillbirth, miscarriage, cesarean birth, or complications during pregnancy or delivery. If you find yourself having big feelings about your delivery, thinking about it a lot, feeling like a failure, or experiencing mood changes when it comes up, part of your healing should include unpacking your birth story. One way you can do this is to ask a trusted person to listen without judgment to your entire birth story. Seek professional mental health counseling to determine if you have perinatal or postpartum PTSD and receive treatment. Use them as a sounding board to talk about the parts of your experience that most affected your core beliefs about your life, your strengths and weaknesses, your spiritual beliefs, your value as a person, and your ability to believe in new possibilities and recover from your experience. Ask your ob-gyn or midwife provider to explain the purpose of something that happened for more understanding. Journal your story and how you felt about it. Hire a postpartum doula.

For a more esoteric approach, read and follow Tami Lynn Kent's *Mothering from Your Center*, which teaches you how to walk through your birth story and reclaim your entire birth field and energetic connection to yourself and your child. One of our interviewees found help with David Grand's *Brainspotting*, an offshoot of eye movement desensitization and reprocessing (EMDR), which uses fixed eye positions to assist in healing and processing trauma.

Recovery Kits

You may be inflamed, itchy, road-rashy, and irritated, particularly *down there*. The first poop, as we mentioned, and maybe even the first few weeks of pooping, may require additional supplies. Use a bidet, peri bottle, wet wipes, and anything cooling that reduces wiping and improves inflammation. Don't forget the Squatty Potty or other device that gets your knees higher than hips. Your pelvic floor will thank you. For some, the inflammation is too much to tolerate the elevated knee position in the first week. That's okay. Put your feet on the floor until things are a bit cooled down.

Use cooling pads to soothe pelvic inflammation. Two months postpartum, Ruth was a bridesmaid. In addition to the granny panties and giant pad under the dress (still bleeding), people's comments about her visible panty line (rude!), and the need to pump in her auntie's car during the bridal shower (public nursing wasn't as accepted then as it is now), her pelvis was so inflamed that her fellow bridesmaids nicknamed it the "Hot Muffin" when they got too close during photos.

Today's Ruth wishes she could have given her postpartum self this recipe for soothing, cooling Padsicles (page 38). Do yourself a favor and stick a dozen of these in the freezer a few weeks before your due date.

We recommend using only unscented products near or in your vagina/genitals. Please don't do anything that can introduce bacteria into healing soft tissue or disrupt the delicate and important microbiome, such as essential oils or herbal infusions applied internally. Ruth and the women's health team she works with recommend only lidocaine spray, aloe vera (no alcohol), witch hazel (no alcohol), and coconut oil.

For the rest of your body, we've enjoyed giving and receiving hemorrhoid cream, cooling breast/chest pads, lanolin, lip balm, hand cream, and bath bombs. We've also heard recommendations for conveniently packaged snacks, herbal teas, chocolate, Earth Mama Organic Nipple

> ### RUTH'S PADSICLES
>
> *Ingredients: Sanitary napkins that you plan to use postpartum (usually the largest ones they sell), 100 percent witch hazel, 100 percent aloe vera gel, aluminum foil, freezer bags.*
>
> 1. Unwrap a sanitary napkin and remove the adhesives.
> 2. Stick the pad to a large piece of aluminum foil, open all the way, including wings if they have them. (The foil should be larger than the entire pad, as you will wrap the pad with this later.)
> 3. Generously apply the aloe vera gel to the pad, using a clean application tool. This is the part that will become the coolest, so apply well to the places you will want to be the coldest.
> 4. Spray or apply a light layer of witch hazel over the aloe on the pad.
> 5. Rewrap the pad in the foil you placed it on, without squeezing out the aloe and witch hazel. Put in a freezer-safe bag and date. Place in the freezer for up to 1 hour before use. Padsicles will keep for up to six weeks, not longer. If the freezer is too cold, put some in the fridge.
> 6. Take the pad from the fridge/freezer and remove it from the foil. Apply it to your underwear for a cooling experience. Wear it for up to 1 hour, although 20 minutes is sufficient to reduce inflammation without making a mess. (If you are bleeding heavily, the soaked pad's absorption will be lower because of the aloe.)

Butter, nipple shields, bottled water, straw cups, and Kindred Bravely brand nursing bras. Watch out for herbal teas if lactating—just because something is natural doesn't mean it doesn't pose a risk.

Less tangible items that can ease the postpartum process include home access to twelve-step meetings for postpartum humans in recovery, gift certificates for pelvic health therapy (also known as pelvic floor PT or OT) consults, and massages. Postpartum humans we interviewed also appreciated receiving copies of the books *The Fourth Trimester* by Kimberly Ann

Johnson and *All the Rage: Mothers, Fathers, and the Myth of Equal Partnership* by Darcy Lockman.

EXERCISE

Exercise is awesome for mental and physical health. We'll go into more detail later, but here's an overview of how it can fit into the weeks and months following delivery.

Spend those first six weeks postpartum *resting*. Give your healing tissues time to knit back together and prepare for activity again. You will be busy enough without adding fitness or exercise to your routine. You can plan activity for your body if you need it for your mental health, to lessen stress, and to help you sleep, but think gentle stroll, stretch, or pacing the floor, not walking down three stories and then two city blocks with a baby strapped to you. This basically constitutes a workout, and this is not the time to work out. This is not the time to psych yourself into "getting fit again" or "being ready to return to work." (Those are direct quotes from Ruth's patients, who then injured themselves and delayed their healing as a result.) This is your recovery time. If you overdo it, exercise will be delayed in the long run. This is a short-term recovery cycle that enables a long-term return to activity.

For those with clotting factor disorders, a history of blood clots, deep vein thrombosis, or pulmonary embolism, movement is a part of a multi-step treatment approach. Regular walks, leg exercises, breathing exercises, and position changes can reduce clot risks. The gentle contract/relax cycle of the muscles acts to pump the blood vessels, thereby reducing clot risk. These movements should not include moving very fast, long, or hard, or with extra weight. Notice if any of your movements cause pain and discomfort in the pelvis or abdomen. Reduce time, tension, and effort if they do.

According to Regina Tricamo, LCSW, who specializes in supporting people through their transition to parenthood, pausing exercise can have a real impact on mental health. If you're accustomed to a regular workout schedule, you could experience increased anxiety and/or depression without it. Notice those feelings if they arise and seek support if they interfere with your capacity. In parts 2 and 3, we'll walk you through foundational exercises and get you back to your favorite sports in a healthy way.

A Therapist's Guide to Transitioning to Parenthood, offered by Regina Tricamo, LCSW:

- Acknowledge every change you are experiencing—no minimizing.
- Create open communication with your partner about your needs.
- Meet intimacy needs in nonsexual ways: touch, eye contact, voice.
- If you are not in a safe partnership or are in an uneven partnership, stay safe first and reach out to others second.
- Give yourself grace and time to naturally settle into parenthood.
- Exercise boundaries and give yourself alone time so you don't feel "touched out": use headphones and music, leave the house, close the door between you and your family.
- Get out in nature, even if that means staring out the window, going for a drive, or standing in an open doorway (in safe neighborhoods).
- Trade exercise as your primary means of mental health management with creative pursuits that are more accessible for your body.
- Work on community/support system by paying attention to who offers. Say yes when people offer, giving specific suggestions for your needs and wants. Use long-distance communication tools. Figure out who is local for small helps like being able to get a shower.

CHAPTER 2

Six Weeks

THE SIX-WEEK CHECKUP

Oh, the six-week checkup. It may be the last time you have an appointment focused exclusively on your body and healing (though we want to change that paradigm). It can seem like a lot is riding on this checkup, where you are likely to be given the all clear for things like exercise, sex, and work. With a few tips, you can maximize the effectiveness of this appointment and increase the likelihood of being referred to appropriate care for any dysfunction you may be experiencing.

When Ruth and Courtney had their six-week appointments, they didn't yet know how to get the most out of them. Ruth went to see her usual gynecologist, who had been on vacation during her traumatic birth. Ruth was sore, her stitches were healing, and she wanted to know if her experience during labor and delivery—having to go home with a catheter and a bag of urine strapped to her leg—and her healing were normal. The gynecologist told her that everything was to be expected, Ruth would be fine, and there was no need for an outside referral. The lack of recognition and compassion made Ruth feel gaslighted about what seemed like a traumatic experience.

Ruth found the conversation so off-putting that she didn't see any gynecologist for three years. During this time, she experienced pelvic pain and painful intercourse that she intuited was related to scar tissue from her birth wound. As a physical therapist (PT) with some pelvic health training, she treated her scars with massage and coconut oil and worked on communicating her needs to her supportive spouse. She did pelvic stabilization exercises to stop some sacroiliac joint pain that made rolling in bed painful. Finally, knowing she needed to have a pelvic exam again sooner or later, she made an appointment for a routine exam with the gynecologist who had successfully delivered her baby. This provider confirmed to Ruth that the birth was "one for the record books" and thought it was reasonable to have felt traumatized by the experience. She asked if Ruth was having any incontinence or pain and was delighted to learn that Ruth had knowledge and access to care for her pelvic needs (thanks, Dr. Streeter!). This conversation was a turning point, improving Ruth's confidence and allowing her to release guilt and shame about her birth story.

Courtney's six-week checkup was pretty mundane, other than leaking milk through the front of her T-shirt. She was given the all clear by her midwife, with whom she had developed a close relationship through her pregnancy and delivery. She had a second-degree tear and some stitches, which had apparently healed. She definitely had intrusive thoughts, especially nursing in the middle of the night, but didn't consider herself depressed. Her midwife attempted to insert an IUD, but wasn't successful, so Courtney was put on a low-dose birth control pill, something that wouldn't interfere with nursing, and sent on her way.

The problem was, things really weren't fine. When she nursed, which was all day and all night, now that her milk had come in and she was recovering from her hemorrhage and anemia, it felt like every nerve in her body was on fire. There was musculoskeletal dysfunction, too, like a butt muscle spasm from her first trimester that hadn't ever resolved. Regardless, she started running again, a little, pushing the giant BOB stroller once the baby could safely ride in it. She didn't know yet that a few years down the line, all those little untreated problems would suddenly become big problems.

We've discussed typical postpartum changes and encouraged you to check in with your body. At this point, you may have a small list of things that are still an issue. Before your provider clears you, get answers about the items on that list. If it doesn't happen at that visit, stay in contact with your provider's office through the electronic medical records portal or on the phone. Bring an advocate to your appointment or have them join via video chat or phone call. These issues may be common in the healing timeline, but many of them are also treatable—that is to say, you don't have to suffer hoping they just go away or believing they are the price you pay for pregnancy. Advocate for treatment where you need it. If you are not sure, a consultation or a onetime visit with a specialist can provide insight into your options.

If you live in an area where access to a provider is limited, in this chapter we'll discuss problems that may arise and what you can do about them.

Questions to Ask at Your Checkup

As they say in Passover Seder, for those who don't know what questions to ask, we offer the following questions as suggestions.

QUESTION	FOLLOW-UP QUESTIONS	ACTIONS	ADDITIONAL CONSIDERATIONS
Am I fully healed?	What does fully healed look like?	Consider scheduling a follow-up appointment or ask about a referral to another provider.	Let your provider know what your daily activities are like, including at work and at home. The considerations for a teacher are different from those for a carpenter.
	If I'm not fully healed, what are my next steps?	Referral should be placed and/or home treatment options outlined.	Can you schedule a follow-up for reassessment to ensure you are cleared after more healing has taken place?
	If I'm fully healed, are there any limitations on activities, sex, exercise, etc.?	If there are limitations, ask how they will be addressed, and what the plan is to return to full function.	
Is there still scar tissue?	How long will it take to heal?	Learn what grade (on a scale of 1 to 4) your provider considers your tearing. This will help you to advocate for additional care as needed.	One person's grade 2 tear varies from another person's grade 2 because of differences in medical histories.

QUESTION	FOLLOW-UP QUESTIONS	ACTIONS	ADDITIONAL CONSIDERATIONS
Did you test my pelvic floor strength?		Your provider should ask you to contract and relax your pelvic floor muscles, or Kegel. If you are unable to Kegel and/or are experiencing fecal or urinary urgency or incontinence or pelvic pain, you should be referred to a pelvic health therapist.	Pelvic health therapy is not accessible to all. Chapter 6 of this book provides a walkthrough of pelvic floor exercises and anatomy.
Did you check my abdomen for healing?		Your provider should check your cesarean scar for closure and pain. They can check for a diastasis recti (DR), separation of your abdominal muscles, by asking you to lie down and lift your head. If you have one, ask for a PFPT/OT referral. Typical PTs and OTs are not trained in treating this.	Your abdominal muscles separate during pregnancy, and a weak core can affect your pelvic floor, core, and back. There is more information in this chapter and chapter 8 about DR, a treatable condition.
Are my depressive or anxious thoughts and feelings normal?	Any questions or concerns you may have about your thoughts and mood.	Your provider may have you fill out a postpartum depression/anxiety (PPD/A) questionnaire.	While many postpartum people experience the "baby blues," if these feelings are still present at your six-week appointment, it is more likely PPD/A. Asking for help, including therapy and/or medication as indicated, is a badass move.

QUESTION	FOLLOW-UP QUESTIONS	ACTIONS	ADDITIONAL CONSIDERATIONS
Can I return to intercourse?		A pelvic exam, as unpleasant as that sounds, is the best way to determine readiness for any intimacy, including penetrative sex. *Many people who have cesarean birth can still experience painful intercourse. Method of delivery does not determine penetration comfort.*	The manner of delivery, degree of tearing, progression of healing, and presence of stitches will all be determining factors in your readiness to return to intercourse. Your mental readiness is another important consideration—more on this in chapter 6.
When should I resume birth control?	Which forms of birth control are compatible with lactation, if this is relevant?	Prescription ordered and filled, scheduled for device implantation, consultation for vasectomy if applicable.	Unless you are hoping to become pregnant again right away (not recommended), begin your preferred birth control method before resuming intercourse.
Do I need a referral to a specialist?		This will depend on the results of some of the exams we mentioned above, as well as other concerns you may have.	In addition to pelvic health therapy and mental health support, possible referrals could be for chiropractic services, acupuncture, lactation consultation, nutrition services, and other providers.
Can I return to work?		If you are eligible for Family and Medical Leave, your provider will need to sign off on your return to work.	Be specific about your work duties, including any lifting that you need to do. If you are healing more slowly than anticipated, a pelvic health therapist can also provide feedback about your return to work.

Here are descriptions and definitions of common six-week postpartum conditions that you can check for yourself and discuss with your provider. This information will assist in your self-advocacy and healing and be more educational and accurate than "Dr. Google."

DIASTASIS RECTI (DR)

Diastasis recti is a core muscle dysfunction, in which the six-pack muscle, or the rectus abdominis (RA), has been pulled apart and stretched at the centerline of the stomach, also called the linea alba. Symptoms include bulging or cratering in the center of the stomach when getting out of bed or coughing, back pain, abdominal pain, constipation, and bloating. Your belly can also just look "strange" to you. Sometimes people with diastasis recti complain of still looking pregnant and feeling heavy in the stomach.

The key consideration with diastasis recti is how it affects your body's operation, not your body's appearance. Because of the bikini industrial complex (thanks for coining the term, Emily and Amelia Nagoski) and other body-negative cultural institutions, diastasis recti can be inappropriately pathologized and become a source of obsession and unhappiness. You know your body and should get treatment for conditions that affect your ability to do what you need to do. But remember that your body is always adapting to changes in your lifestyle and environment. Its shape reflects what it is going through. If you never get your linea alba to below 2 centimeters, that's okay. It may have been your lifelong normal, and you never noticed it before. As always, if you are concerned, get checked out by a trusted professional who is qualified to diagnose and treat you.

It's totally appropriate to seek treatment for DR if it's affecting your life. About a third of first-time postpartum humans will have a DR that

---

How to Check for a DR on Your Own

1. Lie down on your back with your knees bent.
2. Exhale, lift your head off the floor, and hold it up.
3. Starting at the central line of the lower ribs (infrasternal angle), use your fingers to push at the linea alba from the ribs to the pubic bone and feel for any craters or separation between the rectus abdominis (six-pack).
4. See how many of your fingers fit laterally into a groove.
5. See how deeply your fingers sink into the linea alba and the abdominal connective tissue; use your knuckles as your unit of measurement.
6. You will end up with two numbers: width, measured in fingers, and depth, measured in knuckles.

You can also note where the DR begins along the abdominal wall: starting at the ribs, around the belly button only, below the belly button, or the whole length of the abdominal wall.

---

lingers past twelve months. DR may be predictive of other dysfunctions, such as back pain, pelvic organ prolapse, and incontinence; some studies show a correlation, while others don't. In chapter 8, we'll cover some tips on how to treat DR yourself, in the event that a pelvic health therapist isn't accessible.

CESAREAN BIRTH SCARS

If you have had a cesarean birth for any pregnancy, you will have a scar. Straining your scar can set you back to the first level of healing and start the process all over again. Following your provider's advice regarding activity level will support your recuperation in terms of time, the appearance of the scar, the pain associated with the scar, and core dysfunction.

Monitoring your overall health is critical now, because mortality rates are high during the postpartum period, and higher for people who have had a cesarean birth. Check for signs of a urinary tract infection—which is more likely because you had a catheter—by smelling your lochia. It should not smell rotten, or like something turned bad. Take your temperature regularly to monitor for a fever, a classic sign of infection. Look at your scar daily for signs of swelling, discharge, increasing redness that doesn't resolve over time, or reseparation.

Activity Modification Recommendations

Does this sound familiar?

> *Lifting is bad! Don't do it! Except . . . lift the baby for feeding and caring! Take the baby to a multitude of appointments over the next six weeks! Put the baby in an extremely heavy car seat and carry this with you everywhere you go!*

Research into activity restriction following a cesarean birth is outdated, and recommendations are anecdotal, inconsistent, and implausible. Here are ones that we can confidently offer:

- Roll into and out of bed. Keep your knees and elbows tucked in like you are in an aisle seat on the plane and don't want that metal cart to take you out.

- Breathe with a sigh and exhale every time you move to reduce pressure in the abdominopelvic cavity and to avoid putting more pressure on your scar.

- Keep a pillow nearby for when you cough/sneeze, particularly during the first four weeks. Hug this pillow to the scar as tightly as you can before you cough/sneeze to reduce pain caused by increased intra-abdominal pressure (IAP).

* Get a heating pad that you can plug in or microwave to a gentle temperature to reduce your pain.

* To move from sitting to lying down or vice versa, roll to your side first. Don't jackknife (sitting up from lying flat or lying down from sitting straight up), which puts pressure on the rectus abdominis and can set you back in your healing. Use your legs as a pendulum by getting them off the bed first and pushing yourself up with your arms. If you get stuck, don't let someone pull on your arms. This will cause you to hold your breath and bear down anyway, right into that scar. Have someone hold your ribs under your armpits and tilt you up using momentum and your body weight.

* Take stairs one at a time and limit the time you spend going up and down them, or take them sideways.

* Move the tiny human from place to place by using a snap-in-place stroller, by carrying them in your arms or a sling, or by using another safe baby-wearing method. Please don't carry the baby in their car seat slung over one arm like a picnic basket! We see this all the time, but it can truly put a lot of stress on your body. Stroller and car seat management is a great job for your partner or another loved one.

Our earnest plea to the medical and insurance industries is to supply and cover community nursing that supports newborn health without breaking the bodies of the humans who gave birth to them. Maybe someday this country will offer paid parental leave to allow postpartum people to rest and heal and their partners to do the literal heavy lifting. A cesarean birth is a significant abdominal surgery and requires ample recovery time. Lean on your support team during this time.

We know that you might not be able to follow every recommendation for rest, healing, and (not) lifting. As with everything, listen to your body. Lochia, the bloody discharge your uterus will shed for four to six weeks, is a good indicator of your effort versus your healing. If any activity causes an increase in bleeding, swelling, or pain, that is a definite sign to rest and scale back.

Cesarean Birth Scar Aftercare

After the wound has closed and is in the remodeling phase, the scar can be massaged, stretched, wiggled, pushed on, and touched. This is tricky, because how can you tell when it is ready? Remodeling looks firmer, holds tighter together, and doesn't make you vomit when you push on it or rub up against it. Start out light, using different materials like a washcloth, a piece of silk, a feather, a brush, or your fingers against your scar for 1 to 5 minutes every day to reduce its sensitivity. Increase the pressure gradually as your tolerance improves. Gentle stretching and touching are safer than a hard sneeze, lifting, or jackknifing. Your nerves will be angry with you at first! Scar pain is like white-hot lightning, itching, or burning. Hang in there. Your future in jeans depends on it.

Scar appearance can tell a story about health and healing. However, a scar can look closed and still not move well. Movement of this scar is important because it attaches to so many layers of muscle that will eventually need to slide (that's what the abs do) to help the uterus and the abdominal wall achieve peak performance.

At six weeks, you can probably wiggle the scar side to side, up and down, and in small circles with your fingers to promote healing. Stop any time the scar looks like it could split again or if there are signs of infection. Massage it to help its layers slide over one another. Massaging with vitamin E oil or applying silicone scar sheets can diminish its appearance. (If using silicone sheets, please follow directions for wear times and removal if sweating.)

VAGINAL/GENITAL BIRTH TEARS AND EPISIOTOMY SCARS

The entire pelvic floor structure stretches a lot during a vaginal/genital delivery. Sometimes, especially during first deliveries, this results in tearing. Other birth conditions, such as the size and position of the baby, interventions such as vacuum or forceps, or a quick second stage of labor can also increase the likelihood of tearing or an episiotomy.

Considerations for Healing a Tear or Episiotomy

CONSIDERATION	WHAT TO KNOW	HOW TO HELP	OTHER INFORMATION
Pooping	• This might really suck for a while.	• Regular hydration and nutrition. • Possible use of a stool softener or magnesium—ask your provider. • Knees should be higher than hips on the toilet. • Do not strain! • Rinse rather than wipe.	• Witch hazel pads are cooling and soothe irritated perianal tissue. • Get medical support if there is a tear in the anal sphincter—you may benefit from a prescription cream.
Perineal/vaginal/genital scar healing	• Do not touch it for three days while it is working to close itself. • For twelve days, it is working to regrow tissue. Do not pull on it or do Kegels until the scar gets stiff and can hold itself together without bleeding or splitting.	• Gentle movement and massage in the remodeling stage. • Coconut oil, applied externally at first and then internally at night. • Gentle Kegels and reverse Kegels (page 156) to help the scar work with your muscles. • No heavy lifting.	• A dilator, small vibrator, or finger can be used to gently stretch the vaginal/genital opening after eight weeks or clearance from a medical professional. • Gently pulling the labia or buttocks can do the same.

Considerations for Healing a Tear or Episiotomy

CONSIDERATION	WHAT TO KNOW	HOW TO HELP	OTHER INFORMATION
Infection prevention	• Be concerned if your tear is painful to the touch or emits a foul odor or pus (yellow or green), or if you have a fever.	• Evaluate yourself regularly using a mirror and seek medical attention if you believe you have an infection.	• Let your provider know if your stitches haven't dissolved by your six-week appointment.
Return to intercourse	• Tearing and scarring should be fully healed and evaluated by your provider before you attempt.	• Start slowly. • Communicate clearly. • Focus on arousal as a first priority. • LUBRICATE.	• See chapter 6, "The Pelvic Floor," for more detailed information!

YOUR FIRST PERIOD

After four weeks, the uterus should be done shedding lochia. At six weeks, if you are not working on eight to twelve pumps or breastfeedings/chestfeedings per day, your estrogen may return, causing you to ovulate and have your first postpartum period. If you are lactating or breastfeeding/chestfeeding exclusively and maintaining a strong supply and regular milk expression, you will not have your period for some time. No one can say for sure how many feeds per day will stop your period, and exactly when it might return. We do know that ovulation will occur first, which is why it's important to talk with your doctor about contraception options if you return to sexual activity and don't want to risk pregnancy.

Ruth's first postpartum period was a shock. She had just finished shedding her lochia, and seemingly days later, there it was. She called her best friend, who answered the phone with a cheery "Hello!" Ruth then went into a ten-minute rant about the content and amount of blood she was losing and the unfairness of not being able to use a tampon for it, only to find out that it was her best friend's husband on the other end. He had answered the phone for his wife and didn't have the heart to interrupt. He finally passed the phone on to the right person, who laughed and laughed about the boundaries of best friends with husbands and wives.

After thirty-seven weeks of gestation, the uterus will be expanded. An expanded uterus has more surface area to grow more endometrial lining, which equates to more lining that sheds during your period. That first postpartum period can rival your first postpartum poop for intensity. It can be heavier and crampier, and come with mood swings you haven't felt for ten months. The good news is that these heavier periods tend to resolve instead of becoming your new normal.

Many people do not tolerate tampons for their first period, like Ruth. This may be the case if you had a vaginal/genital birth with tearing, episiotomy, or levator hiatus, a separation of the pelvic floor caused by vaginal/genital birth trauma. You may need to use pads or period underwear. Once your tissues and pelvic floor have healed, you should be able to return to tampon use with comfort.

Menstrual cup/disc users often find that they don't know what to use, since many companies market different models for use before a first pregnancy and after. While there is some utility to this, it also perpetuates the idea that all vaginas and pelvic floors lose shape and structure after pregnancy, which is a gross misrepresentation. You may be postpartum, and you may have heavier periods, but you may find that the larger-size cup doesn't work for you.

Deciding what cup or disc is right may require trial and error, or research on websites such as periodnirvana.com or putacupinit.com. There you can find charts comparing firmness, length, width, and capacity, and quizzes asking about cervix height, period heaviness, activity level, and sensitivities to the cup ingredients.

Menstrual cups have come a long way. There are models designed for a low cervix, some with no stem (useful if you sustained a labia laceration in birth), and some with suction release for those with a high cervix or mobility issues that make removal difficult. All menstrual cups work by suctioning to the cervix, so they leak if you have a tipped uterus, or overt pelvic organ prolapse. Discs sit high in the vaginal/genital canal and rely on vaginal/genital tone to hold them in place, much like a pessary or a diaphragm, making them easier to use for folks with prolapse, but not for those with a high cervix. Despite some interesting Reddit threads to the contrary, there is no clinical evidence that use of a menstrual cup leads to prolapse. If you have good to high pelvic floor tension, make sure you get a cup that is on the firmer side, so it doesn't accidentally lose suction when you Kegel or exercise.

VAGINAL/GENITAL DRYNESS

Vaginal/genital dryness can feel like itching and occur when you're just going about your day. Especially if you're lactating, it is to be expected. It can also occur during intimacy and seem like lack of arousal. (See chapter 6 for a deeper dive into this important topic.) Possible daily treatment options include coconut oil or a moisturizing product like Medicine Mama's Apothecary Vmagic or Replens, and of course lubrication during intercourse in particular is key.

RETURN TO MOVEMENT

Once you're cleared to exercise at your six-week checkup, that does not mean exerting yourself at your prior level, even if you exercised throughout the pregnancy. In part 2, we will walk you through returning to movement and exercise while reducing risks like incontinence, pelvic girdle pain, and prolapse, but the short answer is to start with easy, short sessions and rebuild your foundational strength first.

The best reasons to return to any physical activity, whether you want to call it exercise or not, are improved mood, assistance in managing symptoms of anxiety and depression, better sleep, and cardiovascular fitness. *Please note we did not say weight loss. Your worth and healing are not based on a number on a scale.* Focus on other markers of health: how you feel, sleep, care for yourself, engage in activities that bring you joy, and complete the tasks you need to live your life or do your work in the world. These are the places many of us find meaning, and exercise and physical activity can help get us there. Make that the focus of any physical activity instead of punishing your body for having been pregnant or eating.

Postpartum Healthcare

While we hope this book will help you attain optimal postpartum health, it is not a replacement for personalized healthcare. Understanding *how* to get to care is a key driver in getting what you need. In this chapter, we'll guide you through the confusing system of who can treat you for specific issues and how to get referrals, and help you understand what your insurance will cover. We'll educate you on health inequities caused by lack of universal healthcare and explain how services supposedly covered by insurance affect your out-of-pocket costs. We'll also address issues with healthcare bias related to race, gender, sexual orientation, socioeconomics, and geographical proximity to care.

Pelvic health therapy, provided by a physical or occupational therapist, plays a vital role in evaluating, treating, and managing a variety of typical issues, yet many people don't know it exists! We will teach you how to differentiate pelvic health PT/OT from conventional care. You'll also learn how to acquire a referral, what to expect at the first visit (it's not all about Kegels), and how to advocate for trauma-informed care, gender-affirming care, and medical consent.

POSTPARTUM EMERGENCIES

America has an ongoing, and worsening, crisis in maternal mortality and morbidity. CDC data reveals an increase from 17 to 24 maternal deaths per 100,000 live births between 2017 and 2020. The numbers are heartbreakingly worse when broken down by race, with a maternal mortality rate of 55.3 per 100,000 live births for non-Hispanic Black women.

The reason for America's shameful maternal mortality rate—the highest of any developed nation—has a lot to do with our cultural focus on the baby rather than on the pregnant person, as well as factors related to systemic racism and biases, complicated by age, education, geographic

58

location, housing security, mood disorders, poverty, access to transportation, and addiction. According to Dr. Damali M. Campbell-Oparaji, MD, an assistant professor and board-certified ob-gyn at Rutgers New Jersey Medical School Department of Obstetrics, Gynecology, and Reproductive Health, this has led to an increase in complaints of serious medical concerns being ignored or dismissed. Dr. Lisa Gittens-Williams, MD, also at Rutgers, describes this as the "three D's" of ineffective care: denial, delay, and dismissal.

The most common causes of maternal postpartum death are from disorders related to gestational high blood pressure, such as preeclampsia and eclampsia. If you experienced these complications or gestational diabetes, they don't necessarily disappear as soon as your pregnancy ends—and they increase your lifetime risk for cardiovascular disease and other comorbidities (as does just being pregnant). Having a COVID-19 infection during pregnancy, particularly a moderate to serious one, also increases the risk of hypertensive disorders and associated cardiovascular disease. Having this information allows you or your advocate to effectively communicate with your provider, especially in the event of a medical emergency.

If, within the first year postpartum, you experience symptoms such as:

- headaches that won't go away or that get worse
- dizziness or fainting
- changes to your vision
- fevers of higher than 100.4 degrees
- swelling of your face and/or hands
- difficulty breathing
- nausea and/or vomiting, belly pain
- chest pain

treat it as an emergency. The CDC's Hear Her campaign offers a script that you and/or your advocate can use to talk to whatever provider you see in order to ensure they're aware that you're postpartum and should consider that in your treatment. If you're admitted to an emergency department, communicate this information to any provider, technician, or nurse you see.

Postpartum psychosis is a rare but serious mental health condition that can arise within the first year after pregnancy, often in people with a personal or family history of psychosis or bipolar disorder. It's defined as a break with reality, and symptoms can include hallucinations, irrational thoughts or paranoia, irritability, sleeplessness, and a flat affect. Maternal death by suicide occurs in 5 percent of postpartum psychosis cases, and infanticide occurs in 4 percent; postpartum psychosis should be regarded as a true emergency. You or a member of your trusted network should call your provider or emergency services should any of those symptoms occur.

Other Pregnancy-Related Health Conditions That Need Medical Attention

CONDITION	RISK	CALL YOUR PROVIDER IF . . .
Diabetes	Seven times higher if you had gestational diabetes	You notice increased thirst, urination, exhaustion, or rapid and unexplained weight loss.
Clotting disorders	Increased six to eight weeks postpartum	You have a fever; you feel warm, painful, and swollen areas of your legs; or you experience shortness of breath or chest pain.
Sepsis	Sepsis is the second leading cause of pregnancy-related death. Risk is increased if you: • Have diabetes • Had invasive procedures to assist fertility • Had invasive tests during pregnancy • Are Black	The Sepsis Alliance uses this mnemonic: • T—increased temperature • I—infection • M—mental decline • E—extremely ill

Other Pregnancy-Related Health Conditions
That Need Medical Attention

CONDITION	RISK	CALL YOUR PROVIDER IF . . .
Peripartum cardiomyopathy	Occurs rarely (10/10,000 births). Risk is increased if you: • Are older or younger than average • Have had three or more pregnancies • Carried twins • Use cocaine • Are Black	• You feel breathless when you lie down. • You are awakened by the feeling of breathlessness after one to two hours of sleep.
Myocardial infarction (MI)	Increased during and after pregnancy	You experience chest pain.
Stroke	Occurs in 30/100,000 births, but risk increases to 1/500 if you had preeclampsia. Risk also increases if you: • Have migraines • Have vascular conditions • Have lupus • Have chronic kidney disease • Were diagnosed with high blood pressure before becoming pregnant • Had gestational diabetes • Had a cesarean birth	You experience any of the following: • Sudden one-sided numbness or weakness in face, arms, or legs • Dizziness and difficulty walking • Loss of vision • A sudden severe headache • Slurred speech
Breast cancer	Increased within five years of giving birth	It can be difficult to differentiate typical changes in breast/chest tissue after birth from changes due to cancer. Discharge, pain, an itchy rash around your nipple, and redness or darkness of the skin should be monitored. The most concerning symptom is a new *painless* mass in the breast/chest.

Where you live can radically alter the likelihood of receiving appropriate care in an emergency. The nearest hospital may not have the ability to treat you, which is something to consider if you have risk factors. Coordination of care and insurance coverage vary from state to state as well. Some have implemented legislation or other programs to improve maternal outcomes in response to the CDC data, such as a Medicaid expansion to allow for coverage for a full year postpartum, rather than the standard six to eight weeks. Some participate in the Alliance for Innovation on Maternal Health (AIM), which allows for a coordinated response to maternal health crises, including cardiovascular and hypertensive emergencies. However, there isn't yet a federal-level plan to make sure pre- and postpartum health concerns are taken seriously.

ACCESSING HEALTHCARE

The goal of seeing a healthcare provider is to shorten your healing timeline, prevent disability, and meet your specific health and wellness needs. The outcome should be you feeling better than you did and understanding how to manage your health condition. If you want to see your primary care physician (PCP), gynecologist, or midwife, you are already established in those offices and can call at any time to set up an appointment. Some offices will have you first meet or speak with a nurse or a mid-level provider like a physician's assistant (PA) or family nurse practitioner (FNP), who will triage any "new" issues. Who you see will depend on who is available and how that office handles "new" issues.

You may find that you need non-physician-level services or support services for your postpartum recovery, including physical or occupational therapy, chiropractic, osteopathy, acupuncture, massage therapy, counseling services, postpartum doula services, and nutrition counseling. Any of the above can help you heal beyond the medication, surgery, injections, or diagnostics you would get from a regular physician.

Knowing what services you need, finding providers, and getting to them can be difficult, especially in a postpartum haze. Most of the providers listed below will see you at least once for a consultation and determine from there if you need additional care. Ideally, you will be able to pick and choose from available services based on your needs, find the most appropriate providers, and make the best investment of your time and financial ability in your recovery.

What Services Do I Need?

These services could be available based on where you live. Most are covered by insurance in some way, but all will be at the mercy of your deductible, out-of-pocket max, co-pays, and in/out of the network provider status. You should be able to use a health saver or flexible spending account to pay for out-of-pocket costs. Some of them will be better covered by insurance if you have a referral from your PCP, gynecologist, or midwife. Some states will allow direct access to these providers without a referral; facility policies will still dictate the easiest way for you to get an appointment. Speak with the office ahead of time to get correct information for your circumstances.

Postpartum Medical Treatment Options

SERVICE	CONDITIONS TREATED	TREATMENTS PROVIDED
Physical therapy (PT)	Almost any issue with the joints, muscles, ligaments, tendons, nerves, including: • Back pain • Shoulder pain • Neck pain • Hip pain • Symphysis pubis pain • Sacroiliac pain • Sciatica • Difficulty walking • Balance difficulty	• Exercise • Manual therapy • Scar mobilization • Gait training • Balance training • Coordination • Bracing/taping • Education • Electrical stimulation • Ultrasound • Traction • Dry needling • Return to sport/work

Postpartum Medical Treatment Options

SERVICE	CONDITIONS TREATED	TREATMENTS PROVIDED
Occupational therapy (OT)	Issues related to function, including: • Use of your hands, elbows, arms • Inability to perform self-care or work tasks • Carpal tunnel • Tennis or golfer's elbow Issues related to cognitive function, including: • Postpartum depression as it relates to your household or workplace ability • Issues with physical and psychosocial performance of parenting tasks • Issues with rejoining the workplace • Breastfeeding support	• Exercise • Manual therapy • Gait training • Balance training • Coordination • Bracing/taping • Education • Electrical stimulation • Ultrasound • Self-care • Posture • Ergonomics • Return to work
Pelvic floor PT (PFPT) or OT	Issues related to bladder, bowel, and genital health, including: • Diastasis recti • Incontinence • Dysfunctional voiding • Sexual pain • Genital pain • Prolapse • Pelvic girdle pain • Tailbone pain • Constipation • Fecal incontinence	• Lifestyle modifications • Education • Exercise • Manual therapy • Posture • Breathing • Core • Pelvic floor muscle rehabilitation • Visceral mobilization • Scar mobilization • Biofeedback • Bracing/taping • Dry needling • Return to sport/work
Chiropractic	Issues related to spine and joint dysfunction, including: • Symphysis pubis dysfunction or separation • Sacroiliac joint dysfunction • Sciatica • Back pain • Hip pain	• Imaging • Manipulation • Mobilization • Electrical stimulation • Ultrasound • Soft tissue mobilization • Bracing/taping • Home exercise program

Postpartum Medical Treatment Options

SERVICE	CONDITIONS TREATED	TREATMENTS PROVIDED
Chiropractic *(continued)*	• Pelvic girdle pain • Tailbone pain • Rib dysfunction	• Education • Nutrition and lifestyle counseling
Osteopathy	Issues related to spine, joint, and soft tissue dysfunction, including: • Symphysis pubis dysfunction or separation • Sacroiliac joint dysfunction • Sciatica • Back pain • Hip pain • Headaches/neck pain • Pelvic girdle pain • Abdominal pain • Vaginal/genital pain • Tailbone pain	• Manipulation • Mobilization • Soft tissue mobilization • Visceral mobilization • Bracing/taping • Home exercise program • Education • Standard medical care
Acupuncture	Chinese Medicine or Five Elements approach can treat a host of systemic issues, including: • Pain • Muscle spasms • Stress • Headaches • Hormone imbalances • Postpartum depression • Fatigue • GI disorders • Lactation support	• Insertion of acupuncture needles • Acupressure massage • Electrical stimulation • Heat application • Herbs • Aromatherapy • Cupping • Moxibustion • Taping
Massage therapy	Issues related to soft tissue and pain in the fascia, muscles, tendons, ligaments, including: • Pain • Edema • Inflexibility • Spasms • Trigger points • Headaches • Anxiety • Tension • Depression	• Massage of various types • Cranial-sacral techniques • Myofascial release • Taping • Stretching • Aromatherapy

Postpartum Medical Treatment Options

SERVICE	CONDITIONS TREATED	TREATMENTS PROVIDED
Counseling	Issues related to mental and psychological well-being, including: • Postpartum depression • Postpartum anxiety • Traumatic birth • Substance use disorder • PTSD • Psychosocial support for parenting transition • Loss/grief counseling • Medical disability support	• Cognitive behavioral therapy • Brainspotting • Goal setting • Coping with feelings • Solving problems • Learning how to respond to changes in your relationship and body • Relationship help
Postpartum doula	• Infant care/training • Emotional and physical recovery support • Transition to parenting support	• Breast/chestfeeding support • Help with the emotional and physical recovery after birth • Light housekeeping • Running errands • Assistance with newborn care • Light meal preparation • Baby soothing techniques • Sibling care • Referrals to local resources such as parenting classes, pediatricians, lactation support, and support groups

YOUR IDEAL PROVIDER

Your time and money are precious, and that's especially true during the postpartum period. How can you select the best provider for your needs in a way that will honor your bandwidth, funds, transportation needs, schedule, and child-care challenges?

Begin by talking to your doctor. This ensures that any issues you're having are medically documented and managed. This also streamlines the referral process and will direct you toward providers who are known and trusted by your PCP, your gynecologist, or another person who sees you regularly and knows you well.

Referrals are often required by insurance providers and healthcare offices to use your coverage to its maximal benefit. The referral both holds your space at the practice and ensures that insurance will cover the appointment, minus your co-pay or other fees. While your doctor may have someone they recommend, you always have the right to request a referral to the provider of your choice. If, for example, your PCP's office typically refers its patients to a physical therapist with whom your friend had a bad experience, you can request a referral to someone you've heard better things about. Recommendations from your community can help you select the best possible provider when multiple options are available.

What other factors can help you choose from multiple available providers?

1. **Who will cost you the least out of pocket?**

2. **Who best matches your healing style?** Do you prefer as few visits as possible and to be given "homework" to facilitate your healing? Or would you prefer to put your care wholly into someone else's hands? Somewhere in between? Talking to your doctor can guide you toward the best provider for your preferences.

3. **How accessible are they?** Do they have a wait list? Do they work only certain days and certain hours? How easy or difficult will it be to get to their office from your home or workplace?

4. **Who has the most expertise in your area of concern?** Not all providers are postpartum literate. Checking their website, calling their office, and talking to your referring provider can help answer this question.

5. **Who feels like the best fit for you?** Healthcare outcomes are better when we're cared for in ways that are meaningful to us and that affirm our entire selves. You may encounter a provider who doesn't feel right to you. Maybe you don't like their personality or treatment style; maybe your visit felt rushed, and you didn't have all of your questions answered; or maybe you would prefer to have a provider who looks like you or shares life experiences with you. Trust your intuition. You will need to be vulnerable with this person, so a positive patient-provider relationship is vital.

INSURANCE AND THE REFERRAL PROCESS

Conventional Medical Care

If you have insurance (we hope someday that includes everyone), you want to make it pay as much of your healthcare costs as possible. This can be tricky! Once you have a referral for specialist care, follow these steps to make your coverage work for you:

Step 1. Have your referral sent to your preferred provider's office.

Step 2. Call your insurance and find out what the coverage is for that service. You will get these numbers:

Co-pay—This is the amount you will owe per visit to this provider, regardless of how long you are there. This depends on what type of service you are visiting and whether the provider is in or out of your network.

Deductible—This is the amount you will have to pay out of pocket before your insurance will pay for anything. Some insurance plans have a high deductible, and others have their coverage kick in right away. Having a deductible can impact how much you pay depending on the time of year you access service, since everything resets on January 1. This really sucks and can lead to people who enter the postpartum period in the last quarter of the year putting off needed care.

Coinsurance—This is the amount you have to pay per visit after your deductible is met. This is the sneakiest, most ridiculous way insurance companies make money because it is never transparent. The more expensive the visit, the more you will pay.

Out of pocket—This is the amount you have to pay before your insurance coverage matches 100 percent of the cost for a given service (that is to say, no more coinsurance).

Visits per year—While the number of covered visits per year should be "as many as you need," many plans have a preset number of visits for a given service per year for any diagnosis or an authorization method to grant you an arbitrary-seeming number of visits for each diagnosis. On your first visit, your provider may submit an authorization request to the insurance company. Based on the information in the report, the insurance company comes up with the number of authorized visits. The math is totally opaque. Your provider can request reauthorizations if more visits are needed.

Your insurance company will mail or post to your online portal an Explanation of Benefits. This will break down what was billed, what was covered, and how everything has accrued over the year. It's worth reading through (says the person who pretty much just recycles them).

Step 3. Call the office your referral was sent to, confirm that they received it, and schedule the appointment. Ask if they recommend scheduling more than one appointment at a time, and then do it. Ruth's waiting list can be from four to eight weeks. You don't want to wait four weeks between your first and follow-up visits. You can always cancel or reschedule.

Step 4. Ask about the billing process. Do they bill per visit, per time code, or per procedure? Can they provide an estimate? Do they offer payment plans?

Step 5. If you would like and it's available, ask to speak with your provider beforehand. This isn't to obtain treatment over the phone but is a compatibility assessment and a way they can help you understand what they do and what to expect.

Step 6. Get to your appointment. This is often the last barrier. We understand all the factors that have to fall into place for you to make it to your appointment. Time, including possibly time off from work. Transportation. Child care. Vulnerability. Putting one more thing on your plate. Belief that your symptoms are treatable. We just ask that you get to that first visit and give yourself the gift of hope. There are people dedicating their lives to helping you; let them try. You are worth it. (You can usually bring the baby, too.)

Step 7. If you go through steps 1–6 and you aren't seeing improvement, didn't like your provider, or didn't attend your appointment, begin again. Enlist the members of your support community to keep you accountable for making good decisions about your health. Hang in there. There is help. You can heal.

Other Ways to Access Care

What if you don't have insurance or your deductible is high and you still need to access care? Based on the provider you want to see and the laws in your state, you may be able to directly access one. Direct access eliminates the need for a referral and gives you the opportunity to present your health concerns to the clinic you'd like to use. Often these are private clinics or offices, which can have lower billing than hospital-based healthcare providers. Some offices provide free clinic spaces each month, to eliminate financial barriers. They are angels and we love them.

Private practices often set a billing amount per visit, per type of treatment, or per time spent in the office. They might ask you to submit your own claim, as they may not employ someone to handle the paperwork. Your bill could be lower and will definitely be more transparent. However, it requires more legwork on your end—one more thing to add to your plate—and the possibility of "out of network" charges not going toward your "in network" deductible. (More mysterious insurance math!) This is another reason to read your Explanation of Benefits.

PELVIC FLOOR PHYSICAL OR OCCUPATIONAL THERAPY (PFPT/OT)

Of the services we've talked about, pelvic floor or pelvic health therapy are the standouts. Pelvic health therapists are board certified and licensed physical or occupational therapists who have taken further study in the treatment of conditions that affect the pelvic floor, including bladder, bowel, and sexual health issues, prolapse, and pelvic pain. Although other providers may give supportive care for these concerns, only a pelvic floor physical therapist or occupational therapist (PFPT/OT) can directly assess and treat your pelvic floor.

The pelvic floor is a collection of muscles that attach internally to the pelvis. Their job is to hold up your sphincters and internal organs. When you were pregnant, they had the additional job of supporting the increasing weight of a tiny human. Pregnancy is an endurance test for the pelvic floor muscles, and this can lead to pain, injury, and dysfunction. You may have had symptoms of a pelvic floor condition (such as incontinence, constipation, or pelvic pain) that have now more or less resolved. Or you may be surprised to have symptoms following a cesarean birth. You may have sustained an injury during an attempted or completed vaginal/genital delivery.

People are often told to simply do Kegels. But this strengthening exercise is only *one* of the things a pelvic floor must be able to do. It's like asking your hand to only ever make a fist, instead of playing a piano, throwing a ball, or knitting a sock. A healthy pelvic floor is much more than the strength of its Kegel. The muscles require flexibility, coordination, power, and resilience in every position your body gets into and the ability to work with adjoining systems of the body. A pelvic health therapist will assess and treat this, far beyond Kegels.

A PFPT/OT Evaluation

A pelvic health evaluation is not standardized, although it will involve a medical intake including your diagnosis, chief complaint, goals, past medical history, medications, allergies, and surgical history. The therapist will probably make you do a functional outcome assessment—aka the Terrible Questionnaire—to give your symptoms a score that your insurance likes.

The physical part of the evaluation is an examination of your body. Therapists will check the range of motion, strength, sensation, reflexes, posture, walking, and balance related to your problem. Therapists will probably touch your body, and you should tell them if you are uncomfortable with that or need that to happen in a specific way.

The thing that is different about PFPT/OT from any other therapy is that they will ask if they can evaluate your pelvic floor. That probably means removing your pants and underwear and lying on a table with your knees bent. The PT/OT will then look at your external genitals and touch your muscles with gloved and lubricated hands to determine sensation, pain, spasm, range of motion, and strength. They will touch and move scars to assess healing. If this is okay externally, they will determine if they need to check the muscles from inside the vagina/front hole and/or rectum based on your symptoms. This is the standard way to test the pelvic floor muscles for dysfunction. If this sounds or feels outside your comfort zone, there are workarounds, and your therapist can explain your other options and act within your boundaries.

This exam is all about tissue health. Therapists look for muscle health and performance in order to develop a treatment plan tailored to you. They will not be using a speculum. They will not do a PAP smear or be able to tell you if you have an infection or other pathology. You still need to see your PCP or gynecologist for that. If they are concerned about something outside their purview, they will probably recommend you see your regular medical provider for treatment.

This examination does not have to be painful, and it does not have to be completed in the standard way if you don't want it to be. Ruth has done many evaluations in various ways to make sure the patient is comfortable. No matter what level of assessment is carried out, your PFPT/OT should do everything in their power to treat your complaint. They should earn your trust and support your mental and physical health. They should support your communication with other health practitioners you may be seeing to coordinate care. Ruth is famous for drawing treatment plan diagrams for her patients to share with their mental health providers.

Finding a Postpartum and Pelvic Health Provider

Not every community has pelvic health therapy as part of their hospital-based care. Many pelvic health therapists are private clinic owners and might be slightly harder to find. Check out the lists maintained by these organizations:

Herman & Wallace Pelvic Rehabilitation Institute
The APTA-Pelvic Health Section

Core Exercise Solutions' Pregnancy & Postpartum Certified Exercise
Specialist

Julie Wiebe, PT

Pelvic Guru and Global Pelvic Health Alliance, run by Tracy Sher, PT

Vagina Rehab Doctor Women of Color Pelvic Floor PT Directory

Institute for Birth Healing, run by Lynn Schulte, PT

The crucial factor in selecting a provider is that you connect with them. A provider who engages with you in the first session, explains their clinical reasoning, uses compassionate language, teaches and educates without scaring you, works with you to make understandable and achievable goals, and explains the plan can lead to improved health outcomes even before treatment begins. All humans, and perhaps especially postpartum humans, need to be heard and validated. When practitioners provide that level of care and stay curious about your responses, they can adapt to best suit your needs. You'll feel the difference.

POSTPARTUM MENTAL HEALTH

PPD/PPA

Postpartum depression (PPD) is experienced by one in eight birthing parents, according to 2020 findings by the CDC. About 50 percent of people reporting symptoms of depression will go untreated, despite many postpartum people undergoing screening for PPD, often at their baby's pediatric appointments. Most of our interviewees reported being asked about their mental health more frequently than their pelvic health or postpartum pain.

Postpartum depression is not to be confused with the "baby blues," sadness or moodiness following delivery. The baby blues should alleviate within two weeks. PPD, meanwhile, occurs in weeks one to three postpartum and can last for years. It does not get better on its own. PPD is more than fear or anxiety about life and the future or a little sadness. It causes a withdrawal from life and lack of engagement with family members, including a lack of bonding with the baby. It can include sadness, anxiety, and hopelessness. People with postpartum depression may withdraw from the very people who could support them and advocate for them to get help and the care they need. As it progresses, you might notice that simple daily tasks are difficult to complete. PPD is treatable, but asking and advocating for care can take energy that you don't have. Have your supportive partner, friend, or family member with you at follow-up visits to state clearly how much your mood is affecting your level of capacity to engage and be present in your life. We can be experts at appearing well; interviewee AW described smiling through the entire postpartum checkup despite the fact that it took all of her energy to even go to the appointment. Smiling can be a self-defense mechanism against seeming unwell or needing help from strangers.

Likewise, postpartum anxiety (PPA) is more than just being worried. It's a pervasive worry about the future that does not go away and can be linked to generalized anxiety disorder, postpartum panic disorder, obsessive-compulsive disorder, and post-traumatic stress disorder.

Symptoms can include:

* Constant worry
* The feeling that something bad is going to happen
* Racing thoughts
* Disturbances to sleep and appetite
* An inability to sit still
* Physical symptoms including dizziness, hot flashes, and nausea

Both are treatable, and we encourage you to tell your most trusted person about your symptoms and to come with you to an appointment where you can advocate for care.

Getting Help

The best way to get help is to accurately report your symptoms as they are at their worst. You could be having a better day during your appointment, which can undermine what you experience on those days you can't get out of bed or brush your teeth. Be clear that you know your symptoms have been lasting for a while and haven't gone away on their own. Have someone you trust come to the appointment (or video call in) to advocate on your behalf. PPD/PPA is typically treated with medication and counseling. Advocate for what you think might work for you and talk to your loved ones truthfully about what you are feeling. They can access online resources such as Postpartum Support International (postpartum.net) to help support you.

The National Institute of Mental Health recommends that once you begin treatment for PPD/PPA, you should avoid criticizing yourself or judging your feelings and try to do things you used to enjoy, even if they don't sound appealing. Other recommendations include regular physical activity and sleep, consistent nutrition, prioritizing your to-do list, connecting with trusted friends and family, postponing important life decisions until you're feeling better, and avoiding alcohol, nicotine, and drugs. Some of these recommendations might feel unachievable now, so just do your best. Ask your village for what you need, and answer honestly if someone asks if you need anything. Here are a few scripts if you need help finding the words:

- Could you drive me to my appointment? I'm nervous to go by myself and worry that I will back out.

- I'm having trouble taking care of the house, myself, and my family. Would you be willing to hang out or video chat while I take care of some chores?

- It's difficult for me to leave the house. Would you be open to picking up some groceries for me next time you go?

- I don't want to talk about pregnancy or postpartum right now. Can we keep the conversation to other things?

- I appreciate the invitation, but I can't be around drugs and alcohol right now. Can we do something together that doesn't involve them?

NIMH also provides recommendations for the members of your support system so they can help you access mental and physical healthcare; offer patience, understanding, and encouragement; invite you for walks or other activities; encourage you to stick to a treatment plan; and offer transportation to appointments.

Postpartum Recovery from Addiction

Accessing recovery supports can be especially difficult during the postpartum period. If you're participating in meetings through AA, NA, or similar organizations, it may be possible to attend groups via video call or to have a community member organize meetings that occur at your house. There are groups specifically for connecting with other postpartum people in recovery, often through hospitals or other healthcare centers, and others geared toward folks in medication-assisted recovery.

Medical professionals are often guilty of bias and stigma against pregnant and postpartum people who use substances or are in recovery. There are some initiatives, largely at the state level, which are intended to center patients and guide them to a medication-assisted recovery model—for example, MaineMOM—but they are not available everywhere. Ideally, you and your provider will work together to determine how best to support you (and potentially your baby), while maintaining your privacy. This can be built into the way they communicate with you and each other

---

Postpartum Humans: AW

PROBLEM

AW had a scheduled cesarean birth when her breech baby made it clear he was staying put. She coached herself not to have expectations about birthing, but found that her disconnect and the lack of information she had about the surgery and recovery process led to mental and physical challenges in the postpartum period. She was shocked at how painful breastfeeding was and found it difficult to get support for switching to formula and ceasing her lactation. She was unable to wear the baby for several weeks due to her healing incision and couldn't carry his car seat down the stairs from her third-floor Brooklyn walk-up. Getting to and from appointments in Manhattan would have been impossible without the privilege of a supportive and available partner and the money to pay for Ubers. She struggled to bond with the baby, who needed additional care due to his hip dysplasia.

SOLUTION

When her partner returned to work, AW began therapy with a mental health counselor who was postpartum literate. Although it was challenging to prioritize her own needs, she found that "water, sleep, food, sunlight, and moving her body daily" was her favorite therapy advice.

---

while other family members are in the room, the narrative used to explain a prolonged hospital stay for you or your baby, and the management of pain medication in the event of a cesarean birth. Dr. Julia McDonald, a Maine-based family physician who frequently works with patients with substance use disorders, recommends creating a plan with whoever is helping to manage your pregnancy and is your chosen person—partner, doula, friend, parent, etc.—in case you have a cesarean or other significant procedure that would normally involve pain medication. Be clear, concise, and prepared to repeat yourself (or have your advocates repeat themselves on your behalf) to everyone in the room. Protocols around stopping or changing medication-assisted treatments are inconsistent from facility to facility. There are also different schools of thought about whether taking pain medication as prescribed will lead to a relapse in opioid addiction. Ultimately, this is about what is right for you. No matter what you choose, remember that you do not need to discuss your personal medical history or choices with everyone. You can request that your medical team fiercely protects your privacy.

Part 2

...

HEALING
THE POSTPARTUM BODY

Now that we've covered the first six weeks and some of your immediate needs, it's time to talk about resuming movement and building foundational strength. In this section, we will take you through each part of the body that *can be* affected by pregnancy and delivery. For some of you, you will require intervention to return to a state of physical health that allows you to thrive, instead of being one of many postpartum people lamenting what their body used to be able to do.

We cannot say what parts of this section will apply. You have your own body with its own history, needs, and experiences that shape your recovery in such an individual way that we cannot predict every presentation. Thus, this doesn't take the place of individualized medical advice. Seek out care if you have a medical condition, consult with your physician to get clearance to exercise, and ask for a referral to a postpartum certified physical or occupational therapist for individual assessment.

Our goal is to supplement your healing in the face of a systemic healthcare crisis in the United States, where certain physicians, insurers, employers, partners, and family members do not value the birthing person. You need to be your own detective. View each chapter as an exploration of what your body is doing. If you feel confident about some things, check these off your list and see if you can engage with items that feel more challenging. They may be challenging mentally, physically, or emotionally. If you become frustrated, put that item away and move on to something else. Maybe there is a different body system impacting that problem. Sometimes if you circle back, things will become clearer and more easily accessible.

This section starts with the work you can do immediately and then moves into body systems that make more sense to work on as your healing progresses. We are not using a "start at week x" pattern, because you can begin anytime, whether you are week 2 or forty years postpartum. If you are having significant pain and disability, skip to the section you need. You do not need to complete every exercise or activity to have a positive impact on your health. However, we do recommend that you get familiar with each topic if you plan to return to sports, fitness, or exercise. In the medical world, we call this *prehab*. Time spent on small exercises and conditioning reduces your risk of injury and improves your performance in your chosen activity.

How should you plan your exercises? That is up to you, although we never recommend more than once a day. In fact, two to three days a week focusing on one exercise may be all the bandwidth you have. Remember that one exercise is better than zero. You do not have to complete an entire series to effect positive change. Be gentle with yourself. Your first twelve weeks postpartum have many demands on your time, energy, and recovery. Just focusing on our big three—rest, hydration, nutrition—can feel like a full-time job. If you are feeling like these exercises aren't working, check in with the big three first; your body requires them before you can move on to other facets of recovery.

Before you dive into these new exercises, we need to have a conversation about pain. Pain is tricky. It's your brain's interpretation of its environment and your safety in it. This is why you'll hear some people say that pain is "in your head." That is a gross generalization and misleading. They mean that pain is a neural, or brain, process. Our brains are large central processors taking in a lot of information from all body systems and then providing a signal meant to say, *Pay attention.* Pain in the hip doesn't always mean something is torn or tight or even that there is anything wrong with the hip itself. It might mean that your body wants you to pay closer attention to a process or position that the hip is in, particularly if it's regularly painful.

Correcting pain may mean being stable in posture, reducing surrounding muscle spasms, mobilizing your joints, using surrounding muscle systems to better support the area of pain, getting enough rest to fully recover from activity or work, eating enough protein to feed the muscles for the activity they completed, or working on your nervous system so it's not hypervigilant and hyperresponsive to stimuli. Pain might mean that the spinal or peripheral nerve attending that area is being pinched. (This usually is accompanied by tingling or numbness.) Pain could mean your fascial network is overtaxed and locked in a state of high tension in order to make it through your day, resulting in more pressure on pain-sensitive structures. Pain can occur with muscle activation around an area of healing ligaments or scarred tissues. (When you sprain your ankle, for example, one exercise to treat this injury, which we call ankle pumps, causes the ankle to ache, but makes it feel better in the long run.)

The point is, pain is information, and you must decide what to do with it. Ignoring it won't work. Entire professions are dedicated to this idea, so don't feel bad if you don't get it right. Our number one recommendation would be to bring a painful area to the attention of the right medical professionals to ensure nothing is seriously injured or broken and receive individualized medical care. But we wrote this book because of the systemic and cultural reasons you might not be able to do that. So the next best advice is keep moving—with care. People who are able to keep moving by modifying and reducing an activity get better much faster than people who stop all movement or exercise due to pain.

What should you do if you have pain with exercises or activities in part 2? Check in with yourself. Ruth recommends the rule of threes (this is her professional shortcut for a complex pain system, meaning it works often enough, but not always). Try an exercise or activity for three repetitions. If you have pain but it doesn't get worse, it's likely just information that you are working a body area that is tenuous. Your body is saying *be careful*. Give yourself a chance to warm up and keep going. You likely just had stiffness. If you do three reps and you feel the pain worsening in intensity or location, that's a stop sign. Modify it: reduce the range of motion or weight/effort. Try a less challenging position. Try it on the other side first (this can retrain your brain's perception). If it's still painful, come back to that activity another day. Be truthful with yourself. It might have been something you've done with ease before, but don't have the current capacity for. We will give you beginner, intermediate, and advanced progressions. Drop down a level to where you can do the exercise well, but increase the holds, reps, or sets to build endurance.

What if you have pain after an activity? Sometimes that muscle soreness is a natural response to work and it's just fine. Make sure you're hydrated, fed, and sleeping to recover. If it keeps increasing and gets worse on day two, it's likely delayed onset muscle soreness (DOMS), repetitive tendon/muscle injury, or some other musculoskeletal issue. That means your body pushed through the activity, but you worked at a higher threshold than you can easily recover from. Take an active rest day—walk, work another body area, and when you come back to the problem exercises, decrease the time, reps, or workload.

We hope you can find ways to stay hopeful, keep moving, and remember that pain is just information. Try not to catastrophize and limit yourself based on fear without being assessed by a medical professional to determine if something is that level of serious. Do *not* go to Dr. Google to check out your symptoms. If checking in with yourself and modifications are not working, just go to the doctor.

CHAPTER 4

—————•————————————•—————

Breathing

We think of breathing as something that's instinctive and automatic, but that isn't always the case. The anatomy and physiology of the respiratory system, particularly the diaphragm, is involved in nearly every body adaptation that occurred during pregnancy, including posture, digestion, constipation, reflux, how you use your voice, abdominals, pelvic floor, and even mental health. We'll teach you how to use your diaphragm and how you can tell when it's not coordinated with the rest of the core, and we'll give you exercises for optimized inhalation and exhalation to support recovery and healing.

UNDERSTANDING THE RESPIRATORY SYSTEM

"BREATHE."

That word carries a lot of significance. Maybe you were short of breath during the third trimester. You may have been coached to breathe at certain times or in certain ways during labor and delivery. Your partner or advocate might remind you to breathe when someone is disrespecting your choices and you're trying not to tell them where to go. You took a deep breath in while someone listened through a cold stethoscope before you were discharged from the hospital. Your body moves when you breathe—maybe your shoulders rise with an inhale, or your belly expands. An exhale might bring relaxation or resignation. It could be a sigh, as you try to shrug off another slight. You might hold your breath as you watch a baby or a child sleep, reassured by the rise and fall of their belly. Breath is life.

Anatomy and Physiology of the Respiratory System

The respiratory system begins with airways starting from your nose and throat (pharynx), extending down through your voice box (larynx and trachea) into the lungs themselves (bronchi), which are a system of air sacs shaped like a tree (bronchioles and alveoli) and are filled with a detergent-like substance (surfactant) that keeps them open. Air is pumped in and out of the lungs by the structures that surround them, including the thoracic spine, ribs, sternum, collarbones, diaphragm muscle, and rib muscles, and some of your neck and abdominal muscles.

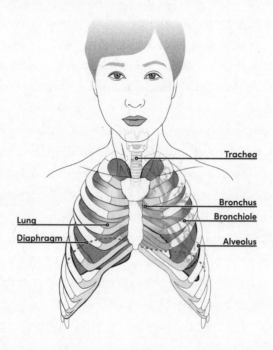

Together, they coordinate to control the flow, rate, and depth of air movement.

Respiration is both involuntary and voluntary. It will happen without your thinking about it, in response to a demand from your organs and tissues for more oxygen, *or* you can take control of the system on your own. The primary purpose of this system is to draw in air rich in oxygen, which suffuses the blood and is pumped to the rest of the body by the cardiovascular system, and to expel metabolic by-products like carbon dioxide (making the lungs an excretory organ, just like your bladder and bowels!).

Any muscle can suffer from imbalance in the postpartum period, resulting in pain, poor coordination, and decreased strength. Returning to peak performance requires a combination of strengthening and retraining the muscles. The diaphragm and the intercostal muscles, those between the ribs, are most relevant to the work of breathing. The diaphragm is the largest muscle of inspiration, located underneath the rib cage, and is typically responsible for 80 percent of our inhalation load. It separates the heart and lungs from the abdominal cavity and digestive organs. The combination of diaphragm and intercostal mobility drives the breath in and out of the body, with activation to lengthen and relaxation to recoil fully, or with the managed pressure needed for vocalization. Using the diaphragm to breathe in when you're at rest, sleeping, or meditating should be effortless. However, this might be more difficult when the shape of the rib cage has changed and you have gotten used to using other muscles to breathe. The intercostals are three layers of muscle living between the ribs. If these muscles have been gripped down or clenched, it can feel difficult or even painful to expand the spaces between the ribs. People notice this after an upper respiratory infection where they are coughing for a week or more. The system can also be thwarted by constant abdominal or pelvic floor tension. Go ahead and try to take a deep breath while tensing up. It doesn't feel very big, does it?

In postpartum people, the respiratory system is affected by changes to the rib cage related to gradual uterine enlargement and hormone-mitigated relaxation of the ligaments. This causes an increase in the diameter of the rib cage (think bra-band size), changing the front angle where the ribs meet, called the infrasternal angle, from 68 degrees to more than 100 degrees. You may be more barrel-chested, with your ribs flipped, flared, or lifted away from the belly. You might have prominent lower ribs where you've never noticed them before. The diaphragm also shifts upward and flattens by four to five millimeters, resulting in decreased functional vital capacity and tidal volume, both measures of how much air you can move into your lungs. Estimates say they return to "normal" at six to eight weeks. Ruth sees many people for whom this is not the case. Effectively, this position makes your diaphragm a little lazy, meaning it doesn't show up to work as much as it did before. Our bodies are smart. They will stay in patterns they are used to, even if those patterns are not helpful! Without intentional retraining, your diaphragm and respiratory system can remain sluggish and inefficient, and you will use accessory muscles of breathing as primary movers instead. You will continue to move oxygen and carbon dioxide as you should, but the secondary function of this system, core support, may be lost.

Do you have seemingly chronic tension in your neck and shoulders? Do you find yourself lifting your shoulders and/or chest with every breath? This is an example of a muscle imbalance in the respiratory system. You have switched from employing your diaphragm and intercostals for breathing to using your scalenes, sternocleidomastoids, and trapezius.

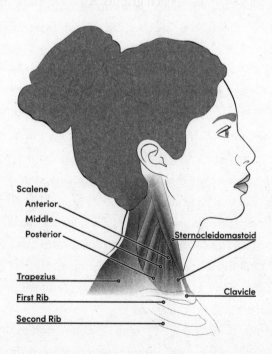

These muscles lift the ribs, sternum, and clavicles up on the inhale and drop them down on the exhale. This is an "inhale up, exhale down" pattern. Since you take an average of 20,000 breaths a day, your neck and shoulder muscles are getting quite a workout! Could this be why you seem never to be able to relax your shoulders and your upper back is always tight? There could be other factors at play, including posture, strength, muscle length, joint mobility, and the use of your body throughout the day. But those breaths aren't helping. They also aren't allowing your diaphragm to perform a vital function: to connect with your deep core system, which includes the abdominals (abs), the back muscles, and the pelvic floor. This deep core system is designed to create and manage thoracic, abdominal, and pelvic pressure to keep you stable in your daily movements and activities. People who inhale up are much more likely to lock their throat, close their glottis, and strain through activities rather than breathe through them. This creates high pressure in the trunk. Repetitive or heavy use of this strategy contributes to a host of medical complaints, including hernias, hemorrhoids, herniated discs, prolapse, and incontinence.

A diaphragm-led breath focuses on inhaling *down* and exhaling up. Most people are confused by this. They have conflated the lifting of the ribs with the filling of the lungs via a diaphragm contraction. The lungs by themselves are not muscular. They rely on something to change the pressure in the thoracic cavity, thereby moving air in/out like an accordion. The intrathoracic space that the lungs inhabit is lengthened by a downward excursion of the diaphragm toward the abdominal cavity. This is the same action used to fill a syringe—nature abhors a vacuum! The movement of the diaphragm down, along with lower, lateral, and back rib expansion, creates the most thoracic expansion and drives the largest breath. With a maximal breath, you *will* see the upper ribs, sternum, and clavicles lift, but we aren't breathing at the maximum volume all the time, and the diaphragm should move *first*.

The rib lifting from "inhale up, exhale down" forces us to use other strategies to exhale, like clenching our external obliques, intercostals, and pectorals or slouching our ribs and thoracic spine, compressing the diaphragm forcefully onto the abdominal contents. You can read more about the external obliques in chapter 8. The external obliques pull the infrasternal angle together and can cause downward intra-abdominal pressure—the pelvic organs and pelvic floor descend—if unmatched by the internal obliques, similar to what happens with bearing down on the toilet. This is the basis for stress urinary incontinence. In order to clean out our lungs with a cough, laugh, or sneeze, we need to pressurize them. If the diaphragm is weak and you then use the slouch/strain strategy to exhale—poof! The core no longer holds you up and in to keep you stable. Instead, it drops down and out, sometimes with leaky consequences.

Recalibrating your respiratory system—that is to say, regularly getting the diaphragm down on inhalation and up on exhalation, what Ruth calls the "blow up!" technique—is crucial for pressure management. This will move the diaphragm, abdominals, and pelvic floor (the core) upward. The rib cage should remain in place without lifting or slouching. Initiating a forceful exhalation through the core is one of the best ways to reduce common postpartum symptoms of urinary leakage with cough/laugh/sneeze (all forceful exhalations) and position change. You may need to say to yourself, *Inhale down, blow up!* multiple times until your body starts to get it. The benefits of this form of breathing will be clear.

RECLAIMING YOUR DIAPHRAGMATIC BREATHING

To take an inhalation breath using your diaphragm:

1. Sit in a chair. It should have a hard surface so you can feel your sitz bones, and your feet should be firmly on the floor.
2. Sit so that your rib cage is stacked on top of your pelvis, like a canister.

3. Make sure your lower back is not arched.
4. Relax your shoulder blades, neck, tongue, cheeks, and throat.
5. Place your hands on either side of your lower rib cage, below the nipple line, and hug your ribs on both sides.
6. Inhale slowly through your nose, taking only a 30 percent breath.
7. Exhale through the nose or lightly though the mouth, but with pursed lips, not flat lips.

What should you feel?
On the inhale:

* The diaphragm should descend toward the abdominal cavity and pelvic floor.
* The lower ribs should expand and separate outward in all directions like an umbrella.
* The lower parts of the trunk including the belly, back, and pelvic floor should stretch outward.
* The pelvic floor and core should be relaxed, but stretched from the inside due to increased intra-abdominal pressure (IAP).
* The upper ribs, collarbones, and neck should be soft and not move at all.
* Inhalation with the diaphragm should take about 4 seconds.

On the exhale:

* The diaphragm should lift back up underneath the rib cage (typically a recoil, not active contraction).
* The lower ribs should recoil and shrink back to size.
* The lower trunk should deflate.
* Your posture shouldn't droop to accomplish the breath out.
* The throat should be relaxed.
* The ribs should stay stacked on top of the pelvis.

- The back should stay straight.
- The pelvic floor should recoil back to resting position.
- The exhalation should take 8 seconds, or at least twice as long as the inhalation.

Quiet breathing seems simple, but many people find it challenging. It's easy to become accustomed to elevating the ribs and shoulders when inhaling. You may have been taught to breathe with your "belly," rather than your diaphragm, through exercise class cueing, singing, or playing a wind instrument. A "belly" breath will be more forward and back rather than up and down, missing the total core activation. You may feel uncomfortable allowing softness and relaxation in your abs. It's also tempting to try too hard—to sit too rigidly, with ribs held high and shoulders thrust back, taking the biggest inhale you can. Remember, this is intended to be a relaxed breath, not a work breath, and the work doesn't involve brute strength but retraining and coordinating your muscles. If sitting for this breath doesn't click at first, try another position, like lying on your back or side, sitting with back support, standing, standing with your back partially against the wall for postural support, or positioned on your hands and knees. See what works and stick with that for a while before branching out. Allow space between each breath, between each inhale and exhale. This practice should lower your respiratory rate. If you start to feel light-headed, you're likely going too quickly, using too much effort, or not exhaling long enough.

BENEFITS OF BREATHING

Other than the obvious benefits of increased oxygenation and removal of metabolic waste, diaphragmatic breathing is linked to improvements in various other health factors including reduction of stress hormones like

A Singer Learns to Breathe

Courtney is a singer and a trumpet player, so for a long time, she had a real superiority complex about breathing. She had been trained in belly breathing, a quick in-and-out motion around her navel. In her twenties she noticed that sometimes it felt difficult to take a deep, full breath. She blamed anxiety—she had just been diagnosed with generalized anxiety disorder—and found that Pilates and yoga helped, both being forms of exercise in which she was instructed to coordinate breath with movement.

Years later, when Courtney became pregnant, Ruth noticed that she was breathing in such a way to avoid putting pressure on her bladder. Postpartum, when her bladder problems began, Courtney wondered if her belly breathing could be part of the problem.

The more Courtney learned about the way the diaphragm and "canister" are truly supposed to function, the more she realized her belly-focused breathing was causing her to overuse certain muscles, which could have contributed to her overactive bladder. Through pelvic floor PT, her overly tight, weak pelvic floor learned to relax. She also began regularly stretching the muscles between her vertebrae, so she could allow her ribs and back to expand. It took time and patience, but after a while Courtney was able to feel her pelvic floor and diaphragm descend when she inhaled, and to lift off her bladder when she exhaled for exertion. She was able to feel her whole canister expand, including her back, for those deep inhales, and breathing was no longer something she adjusted to keep her bladder happy. The up-and-down motion of her diaphragm helped tone and stimulate her vagus nerve, which helped with her anxiety. And for singing and playing the trumpet, sometimes belly breathing was still the correct technique—just not all the time, for everything.

cortisol; reduced symptoms of anxiety, depression, and post-traumatic stress disorder (PTSD); improved attention, focus, and executive function; reduced blood pressure; improved heart rate variability; and better sleep quality. Diaphragmatic breathing tones your vagus nerve, which leads to improved emotional regulation, reactivity, expression, empathy, and attachment; improved digestion, including decreased reflux, decreased constipation, decreased risk of rectocele or rectal prolapse, improved pelvic floor muscle coordination and control, and reduced incontinence; and decreased pain.

All that is to say that practicing diaphragmatic breathing will make you feel better. You can breathe anywhere. It won't cost you anything. You don't need equipment. You just need to make it a part of your routine. Breathing is even effective in helping other muscle systems move and support your body, because it's part of the deep core system. If you're not sure how to start healing the many body systems in your trunk, start with breathing.

BREATHING EXERCISES

Square Breathing or Box Breathing

Inhale through your nose over a count of 4 seconds. Hold and do nothing for 4 seconds.

Exhale through your mouth or nose over 4 seconds.

Hold and do nothing (don't inhale again) for 4 seconds. Repeat.

Continue for up to one minute or as needed to calm and recenter your body.

When to use: Use to regulate your breathing without breathing too quickly, or if you find it challenging to regulate your breathing. Box breathing can help you reduce acute feelings of panic. It's also useful for recentering your focus.

Modifications: Reduce holds to 2 or 3 seconds if 4 seconds feels too long.

4-7-8 Breathing

Inhale through your nose over a count of 4 seconds.

Hold the inhale for 7 seconds.

Exhale through your mouth for 8 seconds (you may need a tight lip for slow pressure release to make it to 8 seconds).

Continue for four to eight cycles.

When to use: Use for relaxation, to reduce anxiety, and to improve sleep and rest. This style is most closely linked to yogic breathing, or *pranayama*.

Modifications: Keep your mouth closed on the exhale and make a sighing sound in your throat.

Stacked Breathing

Inhale through your nose.

Hold it as long as possible.

Sip in small breaths through your mouth, a little at a time until you feel a lot of pressure on your diaphragm.

Hold this pressure as long as you can. Try not to let the pressure rise to your throat or cheeks. Hold the pressure in the thorax or abdomen. Stay soft, don't fight it.

When you start to feel like you might burst, exhale through tight lips long and slow. Do not puff the breath out by breaking the seal of your lips. Exhale so fully that you cough at the end as if your lungs are empty and starved for the next breath.

When to use: Use this to stretch and strengthen your breathing muscles, including the diaphragm and intercostals, and to improve your rib recoil. Stacked breathing also improves blood oxygenation, mobilizes mucus and lung snot, and increases the volume of air you inhale. This can be particularly useful in those suffering from long COVID or other illnesses that cause an unproductive cough.

Modifications: Start with a gentle stacking breath, but don't hold the pressure. Exhale firmly. If you can't hold your lips tight on your own, exhale through a straw.

360-Degree Breathing

While sitting or standing, place your hands on your lower ribs.

Focus on sending your inhale outward into the lower ribs, sides, back, and belly and expanding them as far as they can go.

Sigh to exhale, allowing the ribs to recoil.

When to use: Use 360-degree breathing to stretch the intercostal muscles and reduce tension in the upper abdominals.

Modifications: Add resistance to the inhale by wearing a tight belt or exercise band around the ribs. It should be tight enough to feel like a gentle restriction, but still let you get the breath in. Exhale either through your lips or through your nose.

Balloon Breathing

Put a regular- to large-size uninflated latex balloon between your lips.

Hold it with your lips only—no hands and no teeth. The strength of your lips and the coordination of your soft palate and tongue should be controlling your airways (these form another sort of diaphragm or valve).

Inhale through your nose and place your tongue behind your top teeth to stop accidentally pulling air in from the balloon. The inhalation should cause a palpable increase in the volume of your lower abs and pelvic floor. Try not to lift the sternum or clavicles.

Allow your tongue to rest in your lower jaw, and with tight lips, practice blowing up the balloon without losing control of it. You should be able to get three to four breaths into a regular- to large-size balloon. You should focus on keeping the thoracic spine still, instead using pressure from below, near the pelvic floor and abs, to push the air up into the balloon (blow up!). The belly should not bulge with the exhales. If it does, check that you didn't arch your back or inhale with lifted ribs that need to drop to get the air out.

When to use: Use balloon breathing to coordinate and strengthen your diaphragm. This is a good way to test your ability to control pressure with your diaphragm, which might be stuck in a downward pressure pattern if you worked hard to push out a tiny human.

Modifications: Try this exercise in each of the positions going from easiest to most challenging: lying down with hips higher than shoulders, lying down with knees bent, sitting, standing, on hands and knees, and during core exercises like a plank.

Precautions: Do not try this with latex balloons if you are allergic, and be careful if you have asthma or another lung disease. Too much effort here can *create* downward pressure in the organs, which can exacerbate stress urinary incontinence or prolapse.

What to watch out for: This is a high-level breathing exercise. Make sure you can control your throat to stop the air inside the balloon from blowing back into your lungs when you take subsequent breaths. As you progress, this is a great way to get your core to contract as you exhale, following the breath into the balloon. If you have diastasis recti, prolapse, or stress incontinence, this will take more time. Be patient and work with the basics. Ruth typically sees the "inhale up, exhale down" pattern as the main issue. Your diaphragm may also simply be weak and need more practice.

Sss Breathing

While lying on your back with your knees bent and your arms over your head, inhale through your nose.

Exhale completely while making a tight *Sss* sound like a snake.

The volume of the exhale should remain constant, not getting softer as you go.

Try to exhale so completely that you start to feel tension in your ribs and have the urge to cough at the end because your lungs are empty.

When to use: Use *Sss* breathing to strengthen your exhalation and connect your intra-abdominal pressure and core to your exhalation, supporting your organs upward. This can reduce stress urinary incontinence and prolapse symptoms if done correctly in pelvic decompressive postures.

BREATH FOR CONTROL

Breathing is the safest way for you to start rehabilitating your abdominals and pelvic floor. It can also have quick returns in terms of reduced pain, leakage, and heaviness. Below are two practices people can use to keep their body feeling safe and symptom-free.

Blow Before You Go

The phrase "blow before you go" comes from Julie Wiebe, PT, who has pioneered an approach for reintegrating and coordinating your body systems postpartum called Piston Science, or core strategy. "Blow before you go" means initiating an exhale prior to engaging in an activity, then beginning the activity while still exhaling. She insists that you not fully exhale and *then* move. The timing is crucial. "Blow before you go" is a simple cue that can automate your system to be better prepared for tasks without overthinking them. If you were at the gym and ready to lift weights, you would use your training to set yourself up to move that weight safely. However, it's likely that you don't set yourself up in the same way to lift groceries or a laundry basket, leading to pain, heaviness, leaking, or bulging; unnatural movement patterns; or too much pressure on internal organs, discs of the spine, pelvic floor, and healing abdominal tissue. Beginning your exhale and continuing it through a symptomatic task can reduce this pressure and lessen symptoms.

Exhale with Exertion

The other breathing cue popular with PFPTs is to "exhale with exertion." This reminds you to breathe during a given task, while "blow before you go" cues you to initiate the exhale prior. People may have their favorites, but the goal remains reducing symptoms of pelvic floor dysfunction like leakage or pelvic organ pressure using the breath as a driver for control. Exhalations help coordinate deep core support that may be harder to activate during the postpartum period, but timing and proper setup may mean the difference between dry or wet performance.

Which one should you use? Try them out and see which feels best. Use standing up from a regular chair as a test. Sit and "blow before you go," continuing the exhale into standing. What do you notice? Did it feel easier and more supported? Try again with "exhale with exertion." Did they feel different? Does one strategy work better? If you stood from the chair while holding, let's say, a wiggling, fourteen-pound oddly shaped lump with one arm, which strategy allowed you to get up with the least amount of symptoms, like incontinence, pelvic heaviness, pelvic organ prolapse, belly bulging, or back pain? Use that one.

BREATH FOR PAIN RELIEF

Over time, you will be able to do more robust exercises. For now, use inhalation to gently stretch areas of your body that are tender, sore, or scarred. Inhale into the muscles in the belly if you're recovering from a cesarean birth, or into the pelvic floor if you're recovering from a vaginal/genital birth. Allow the pressure from the inhale to expand the tissues. This may take practice or different positions to feel effortless. Lying on your back with pillow supports under the head, neck, shoulders, and knees is easiest and will create the least pressure.

CHAPTER 5

Posture

Did you straighten up when you read the chapter title? Stop that right now. We mean it. Posture is one of those words that feels judgmental. We're just referring to the way someone holds their body, not whether they would graduate from finishing school with honors. Knowing how to hold your body after pregnancy can be the difference between success and frustration. Although working on posture itself does not seem like an opportunity to retrain your body, it is like the "little work"—that is to say, small repetitions spread throughout the day can mean big gains in the long run. If your posture is contributing to a muscle imbalance, or you intend to go into traditional fitness spaces, don't skip this read.

Persistent habits can make muscle healing difficult. The problem is that you've probably gotten used to holding your body like you are still pregnant. It feels *normal*, even if it's not anatomically neutral. There is no internal system saying, *WARNING, you are shortening your back muscles and sticking out your belly again.* In order to change what you're used to, you first must become aware of it. Then you need to pay attention to it and correct it when you find yourself in a maladaptive pattern. That takes energy, but not a ton of energy, which is why we call it the little work.

POSTURAL AWARENESS

If you are not sure about your posture habits, break out the camera, or have someone do it for you. Sit with your feet on the floor and your bottom on a firm surface. Get into a relaxed posture and then into what you think is neutral—whatever that means to you. Take a photo from the back, front, and side. Compare. What curves and tendencies remain in both photos? These are likely places where you are holding tension. Repeat in a standing position. March in place and swing your arms. Stop and stand still. Take the same set of photos.

Sometimes posture habits differ when you are sitting versus when you are standing, and sometimes tendencies stay the same. Not sure what you are seeing? See if your ear, shoulder, and hip line up from the side. Where does your rib cage sit in relation to your pelvis? Is your trunk shorter or longer in the back than the front? Is there a difference from the left to the right side of your body? Look at what bony curves are sharper in the spine, or are the curves gentle without the appearance of a hinge?

Common Postpartum Postural Changes

- Upper back and shoulders rounded forward (kyphosis) and dropped down
- Head forward of the trunk
- Back of the neck is shortened and tense
- Smaller spaces between the ribs
- Ribs widen apart in the front of the body (infrasternal angle)
- Ribs lift up and away from the pubic bone
- Abdomen bulges
- Lower back is pushed forward (lordotic and/or swaybacked)

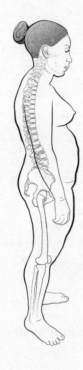
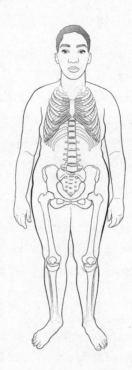

- Pelvis widens and tilts (may tilt forward or backward and may be different when sitting or standing)
- Arches of the feet flatten
- Feet are turned out in standing
- Knees curve toward one another, or too far back

BUILDING ANATOMICAL NEUTRAL

Now that you know what you look like, use that to build anatomical neutral posture. You should always begin from the base of support and stack up from there. Use these cues to practice finding and holding your neutral posture.

Feet:

☐ The feet are shoulder distance apart and pointing straight ahead (check for turnout).

☐ All five toes are relaxed on the floor (not clenched).

☐ The outer heel and ball of the foot are all the way down.

☐ The inner arch of the foot is gently lifted. (This should naturally occur if you did the above.)

Knees:

☐ The knees are stacked over the ankle joint.

☐ The knees are straight, but not locked. (In Maine, we call this *sea legs*.)

☐ The kneecaps should be pointing forward and in line with your toes.

Pelvis:

☐ The pubic bone should be tilted up, supporting the organs (a "seat" for your bladder).

☐ The tailbone/sacrum should gently point down, not be tucked underneath.

☐ The pelvis should be stacked on top of the ankles and knees.

☐ Your pelvic floor, core, and gluteal muscles should be relaxed or gently engaged, not clenched.

☐ The hips should sit evenly in the pelvic socket and be shifted over the arch of the foot and heels (not the toes or ball of the foot).

☐ You should be able to shift your weight from side to side and back to front equally.

Spine:

☐ The trunk is stacked over the pelvis, aligned from the infrasternal angle to the pubic bone in a straight line.

☐ The rib cage sits over the pelvis without leaning left or right, front or back.

- ☐ The spine stays relaxed, not rigid. There is no need to create tension by pulling your belly to your spine, pushing your lower back straight, or pulling your shoulders back.

Head:
- ☐ The head should be stacked over your collarbones, with the ears gently over the shoulders.
- ☐ The chin is relaxed down, and the back of the neck is long.

Seated Modifications:
- ☐ Sit with feet firmly on a flat surface.
- ☐ Sit with weight evenly distributed across right and left pelvic bones.
- ☐ The knees and hips should be flexed to 90 degrees, or with knees slightly lower than the hips.
- ☐ Stack your trunk as otherwise described.

Ruth's Posture Soapbox

Shoulders are not involved in sitting or standing posture. It's time to move past the incorrect notion that cranking the shoulders back and the head up make for "good" posture. Doing this tends to cause too much resting tension in the spine, diaphragm, ribs, voice box, and core that can disconnect you from your pelvic floor. Let the shoulders go free! The shoulders are only a part of posture when you are putting weight on them, as when you are on your hands and knees or are doing planks or pull-ups. True resting shoulder posture is to let them hang. Differences in alignment here, like "forward shoulders," will be due to tension in the body. If your upper trapezius and pectorals are more tense than your serratus anterior and lower traps are strong, then your shoulders will hike up and hang forward. You could appear this way if the ribs and thoracic spine are in a rounded forward posture, which would make your shoulders more of an effect of your posture, not the cause.

TESTING ANATOMICAL NEUTRAL

A good test of anatomical neutral is the diaphragmatic breath. Can you easily practice your quiet breathing in this posture? Does your diaphragm move downward, causing your lower ribs, belly, and pelvic floor to expand? If so, nice job! It can be hard to find the diaphragmatic breath, and sometimes it takes a postural correction to get you there. If you are feeling the breath pull upward to the shoulders and neck on the inhale, scan your body for tension. Whatever your posture at any given time, your effort should match your demand. In other words, just sitting or standing at rest shouldn't cause you to grip or clench any particular muscle group. We're looking at you, butt squeezers and ab clenchers! Try to let the tension in your lower body go and see if that corrects the breath. Alternatively, clench and unclench a few times, wiggle around, and try again to be sure you aren't holding tension without realizing it. Check this posture with different footwear choices and in the chairs you sit in regularly. Try to choose the options that allow you to get that nice posture and an easy diaphragmatic breath. Not all chairs or shoes are created equal, and some can contribute to chronic posture habits that cause pain.

CAR POSTURE

A lot of people, especially those of you with lower back or pelvic pain, feel symptomatic after sitting in the car for more than 30 minutes. Sometimes a lumbar or seat cushion is the answer, but the setup of the car can be the bigger issue. Try these tips to see if you have less pain while driving.

1. **Build from the bottom up.** Make sure the car seat is all the way down and that you can see over the dash comfortably. If not, elevate the seat using the button or lever on the left side of the cushion to where you can see the road enough to safely drive. Depress your brake fully if you have an automatic transmission, or your clutch if you drive a manual.

2. **Bring your seat forward** until you are depressing the pedal fully with a gentle bend to your knee. You should not have to telescope your leg or make it longer to achieve this. Doing so can aggravate your lower back and sacroiliac joints.

3. **Check your tilt angle.** The knees should be at 90 degrees, or just lower than the hips.

4. **Sit up in neutral** without using the seat back.

5. **Adjust the steering column.** Resting hand position is eight and four o'clock on the wheel, with the elbows slightly bent. You can also try the ten and two position, but remember that the elbows should be bent and relaxed, not rigid and straight. Adjust the steering column to sit up straight, holding the wheel, able to see the operator controls, with elbows and shoulders relaxed. Lock the wheel in place.

6. **Bring the seat back up to meet your body** as you sit up in neutral with your hands on the wheel. You should have enough support that you are straight, but not so much that you are being pushed forward—this should feel like a supported slouch.

7. **Check the headrest.** It should be behind the back of your head, not your neck.

8. **Here are some possible alternatives.** You might use a lumbar support if it relaxes your back muscles. Seat cushions are good if you are short and need to see over the wheel, or if you need a cutout for coccyx pain when sitting.

POSTURE TROUBLESHOOTING

The goal is to practice posture as small movement morsels throughout your day until you can hold neutral longer. As your muscles or your body get fatigued, or you get into a task, you will lose it. When you are having pain or notice tension, that's a time to check on yourself. If you are a person who gets sucked into a task, setting alarms or reminders to move every hour can be helpful. Just the sound of an alarm can bring you back to your body for a quick check-in.

Your effort should match your demand. That means that muscles should turn on in relation to how difficult that movement is for you at the time. You do not need maximum activation, clenching, and gripping unless you are doing something strenuous. For some of you, holding neutral might feel strenuous when:

1. **You have a muscle or joint flexibility condition like hypermobility.** This is when the joints are not as tight as they might be (due to injury, disease, or inherited tissue characteristics). Your muscles will have to work harder to hold neutral. Those areas will feel both too mobile and too tight in neutral. Some of you will feel like you just need to pop something to feel better (you probably don't, but your body's receptors might signal that anyway). You might need a support or posture brace or sacroiliac joint belt to stabilize the ligaments so the muscles don't feel they have to work as hard.

2. **You have weakness, and that muscle does have to work a little extra to hold you in place, for a specific length of time.** Usually the longer you hold it, the more aware you are of the strain. Take breaks from being in "neutral" so that you don't end up with muscle spasms. Use back supports and go for walks to break up the posture when you can. We do not recommend using a posture shirt or brace; those will hold you in place, but your body may not learn to hold you there without the support. However, if you are in too much pain, and the brace reduces the pain, that makes the trade-off worthwhile.

3. **You're tired.** When you're tired, your body doesn't have the energy to put into using your muscles in a new way. On those days, it's okay to lean against every supportive surface you can find. Take care of your rest, hydration, and nutrition to allow your body to recover. This is not the moment to push through.

DYNAMIC POSTURE

We have been talking about posture in terms of how you hold your body when you are still or static. The long-term goal of neutral posture is to be able to hold it as you move and perform daily tasks, or have neutral dynamic posture. Here are some ways to check your posture during dynamic activities:

1. When carrying or lifting, load your body evenly. Don't allow the ribs and pelvis to tilt, bend, or shift.
2. When carrying or lifting, use both hands and alternate which side of the body is doing the work.
3. Leaning back when carrying uses more back muscles than core.

4. Leaning forward when carrying uses more core muscles and increases pelvic floor recruitment.

5. When bending to lift, bend all the leg joints together—ankles, knees, and hips—to support neutral spine posture.

6. When sitting, you can cross your legs, but do so evenly. Try to stay in contact with your sitz bones. Alternate sides and stay neutral.

7. Stand without pushing your belly out as if you are still pregnant or sliding the pelvis forward to bear weight more on the ball of the foot. If you do this at the kitchen sink, your shirt will get wet!

8. When standing for more than 10 minutes, have legs wider than shoulder distance apart or one leg in front of the other to reduce fatigue and back strain.

9. When ascending or descending stairs, alternate which leg goes first.

10. When you don't have energy, use supports so you are not slumping your ribs into your belly and crushing your organs down into your pelvis: a pillow behind your back in a chair, a pillow under your arms while reading a book, a nursing pillow to reduce slouching, a head support, an armrest, a footrest.

11. Change positions regularly throughout the day. Any posture held too long can cause pain, even anatomical neutral.

MISALIGNMENT

Misalignment is a catchall phrase used to describe deviations in the body from anatomical neutral. Examples are a tilted pelvis, one leg longer than the other, a sacral torsion, or a rotated spinal segment. It's not a true dysfunction, but it can be an impairment when linked to things like muscle weakness/tension, joint instability/hypomobility, and nerve or soft tissue impingement. Misalignment *doesn't* mean permanent disability. Many people are asymmetric somewhere in their bodies and can live in good health and without pain. Make sure you aren't allowing medical terminology about posture to become a disability if it's not affecting how you live your life. If it is, you might need medical intervention like chiropractic adjustment, osteopathy, physical therapy, or massage therapy.

EXERCISES FOR PAIN-FREE POSTURE

Neutral posture can be tricky to find and maintain if your body feels stuck. This series of exercises can find openness and flexibility in those stuck places and allow you to strengthen your new postures and movement patterns. They should not cause pain. If they do, shorten the range of motion, try fewer reps, or use less weight to make them easier for your body.

Side-Lying Exercises

Rib Rotation

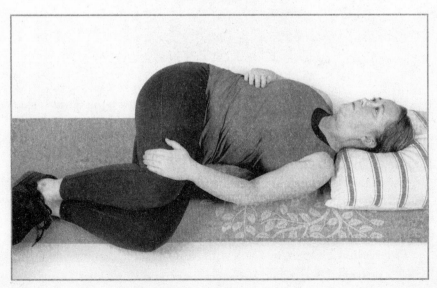

Lie on your side with your knees bent and legs stacked. Place your top hand on your lower ribs. Gently roll your thoracic spine, shoulder, and head back. Keep your pelvis still. This pairs well with a sigh/exhale as you roll to rid the ribs of tension. Roll forward again. Repeat 1 to 10 times. Full range of motion is touching the elbow to the floor as you roll back without moving the pelvis. Having trouble not moving the pelvis? Use the bottom hand to grab the top knee.

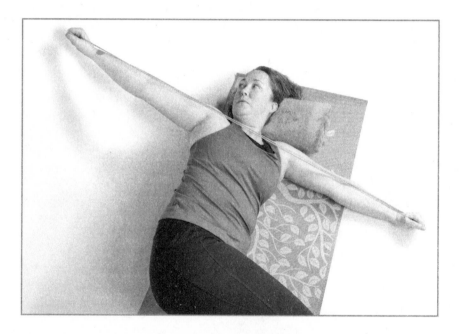

Progression 1. Open the Book or Rainbow: While lying on your side, place your hands together with your elbows straight, hands at eye level. Roll the ribs back, lift the top arm up, align your nose with your thumb as it extends back behind you as far as is comfortable. The bottom arm stays on the floor. Pelvis stays still. Stop when you can no longer roll back with the nose in line with the thumb. Roll forward. Repeat. Full range of motion is the moving arm touching the floor behind you.

Progression 2. Open the Book with Resistance: Repeat Progression 1 using a resistance band held between your hands, or a small dumbbell in the moving arm. Repeat 1 to 10 times. Stop if you lose form to protect your shoulder tendons.

Progression 3. Windmill: Lie on your side with your knees bent and legs stacked. Place your hands together with your elbows straight, hands at eye level. Align your nose with your thumb and lift the top arm up above your head and around behind your body like a large windmill or clock. You should make a full revolution of your arm, up, behind, down, and returning to start. The nose should be in line with the thumb the entire time. The pelvis should remain still. Repeat 1 to 10 times.

Hands and Knees Exercises

Tabletop, aka Neutral Quadruped

Get in a tabletop position on your hands and knees, with your head neutral and the back of the neck long, in line with the rest of the spine. The tops of your feet are comfortably on the ground, with a rolled towel under the ankle if needed. Fingers are spread wide; elbows are straight with elbow creases pointing toward one another. Put your palms on rolled towels or dumbbells if you have wrist pain. Do not round the upper back. You should be able to extend a yardstick from the back of the head along the thoracic spine all the way to the sacrum. This position is neutral quadruped.

Cat/Cow

From neutral quadruped, flex and extend the spine. Cat (flex): push through the hands, round the back up to the ceiling, tuck the chin under, tuck the pelvis under. Shorten the front of the trunk and lengthen the back of the trunk. Cow (extend): sink through straight arms, lengthen the belly (udders hang), sag the shoulder blades, tilt chin forward, stick butt into the air. Repeat 1 to 10 times. No norms for full range of motion here.

Breathing: Exhale with cat (blow up!). Inhale with cow.

Rocking

Hold neutral quadruped and shift your weight forward to your hands without bending your elbows or rounding the upper back. Rock backward, bringing your buttocks toward your heels without tilting your pelvis or rounding your lower back. Focus on keeping a straight spine, pelvis, and elbows. Repeat 1 to 10 times. Full range of motion is sitting back on your heels with good form. Forward shifts can be endurance building if you hold and repeat for 5 to 10 seconds.

Breathing: Exhale with the forward shift. Inhale with the backward shift.

Thoracic Rotation

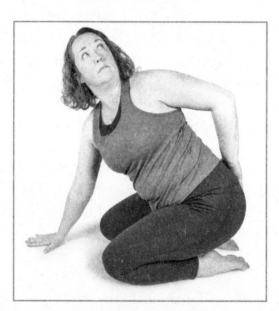

From rock-back position, push into the hand on the floor. The other hand will rotate backward, creating a spinal rotation. The hand can rest on the low back, the ribs, or the head depending on comfort. Repeat 1 to 5 times on each side.

Breathing: Exhale as you rotate. A sigh can help reduce rib tension here.

Child's Pose

From neutral quadruped, rock back until your buttocks are resting as close to the heels as possible. (It's okay to break neutral if the pelvis tilts and the spine flexes.) With your arms reaching forward and straight, lower your torso to the floor, forehead on the floor. Hold 1 to 3 minutes.

Breathing: Inhale to expand the spine, ribs, and pelvic floor. Sigh to exhale and reduce muscle tension. Make sure you aren't belly breathing; this will feel like you are lifting and falling with each breath instead of opening the ribs and spine.

Progression: From child's pose, walk your hands to one side to stretch the side of the body. Keep the pelvis and hips dropped and still. Hold 1 to 3 minutes, breathing as above. Do both sides. If one side is tighter, do an extra set on that side.

Thread the Needle

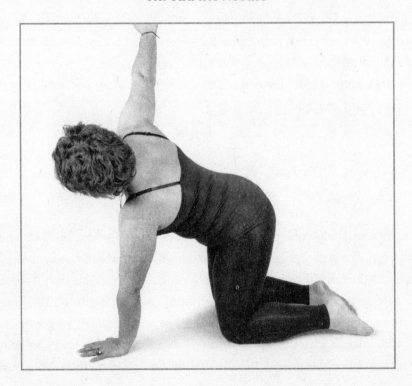

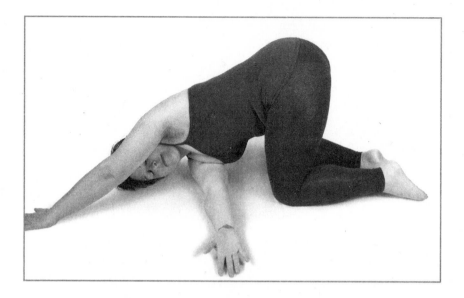

From neutral quadruped, push gently into one hand. Lift the other hand off the ground and reach for the sky as you follow the hand with your eyes and head. Return and reach the hand underneath your body between the planted arm and leg. Repeat 1 to 10 times on each side.

Breathing: Inhale as you reach for the sky. Exhale as you thread your arm beneath your body.

Neutral Lying Exercises

Decompression

Lie on your back with your legs straight. Put enough folded blankets and towels under your upper shoulders and head to allow your lower ribs to come to the floor. The back of the neck should be long. You may have to elevate quite a bit if your back is rounded. The goal is ribs on the floor without force. Put pillows, rolled blankets, or bolsters under your legs until your lower back is comfortable. Alternatively, bend your knees and put your feet flat on the ground. Remain like this for 1 to 10 minutes. Your goal is to lengthen the lower back and rest the spine, reset the rib position, lengthen the psoas, and reduce prolapse pressure.

Progression: Practice the *Sss* or balloon breath from chapter 4 in this position to work on diaphragm and deep core activation.

Arm Exercises

Unless otherwise listed, arm exercises should be done in decompression first, then sitting, then standing. The goal is to hold anatomical neutral and not allow the movement of your arms to move your spine, neck, or pelvis out of position. Arm exercises done in this way, with resistance and proper breathing, double as spine and core strengtheners. You can try "blow before you go" or "exhale with exertion" to build core and pressure management strategies. Make sure you aren't inhaling up. Ruth usually reminds patients to inhale down first and do nothing as you set up, then exhale, blow before you go, or "blow up!" with the pull of the band. The belly should not bulge and the throat should not lock during these exercises. Until you are sure about your ability to hold anatomical neutral, always start from your easiest and least painful posture. Let your effort match the resistance to keep from bearing down or causing muscle spasms.

RESISTANCE BAND/PULLEY EXERCISES

You may be able to use resistance bands at a gym or purchase them online or at a store with a fitness section. Make sure they are designed for the arms, not the legs. If you have a latex allergy, use bands made of a nitrile blend. Resistance bands will break down over time with heat or direct sunlight. These exercises can also be completed isometrically holding a rope, a dog leash, or a yoga strap.

External Rotation

Hold a resistance band between your hands with light tension, shoulder width apart, palm down. Elbows are bent to 90 degrees and next to the ribs. Gently pull the hands apart. Keep the elbows bent and near the ribs, wrists neutral. Return. Repeat 5 to 20 reps.

Breathing: Exhale on the pull. Inhale on the release.

Side Pull

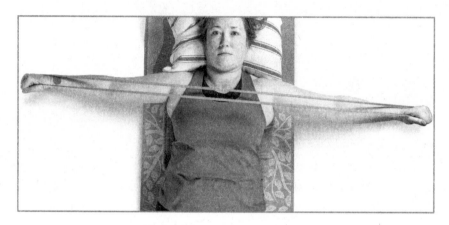

Hold a resistance band between your hands with light tension, shoulder width apart, palm down. Arms are at eye level, or 90 degrees of flexion; elbows are straight. Slowly draw the band apart, keeping the elbows and wrists straight. You should end up in a T. Return. Repeat 5 to 20 reps.

Breathing: Exhale on the pull. Inhale on the release.

Overhead Pull

Hold a resistance band between your hands with light tension, shoulder width apart, palm down. Arms are at eye level or 90 degrees of flexion; elbows are straight. Slowly pull the arms overhead without tilting the pelvis or lifting the ribs up. Release the arms back to the legs. Repeat 5 to 20 reps.

Breathing: Exhale as you lift the arms. Blow up! Inhale as you release.

Pirate Princess

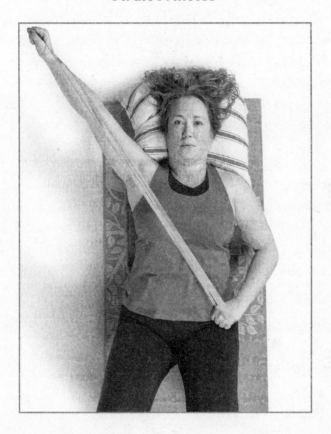

Hold a resistance band between your hands with light tension, shoulder width apart, palm down. Anchor one hand to the pelvis at the side pocket. This is the "scabbard" hand and does not move. Reach the other hand away as if pulling a sword out of a scabbard. It should pass across eye level and land at a 45-degree diagonal above shoulder height as if brandishing a sword. Return the "sword" to the "scabbard." Repeat 5 to 20 times on each side. If you have a noticeably weaker side, do an extra set on that side.

Breathing: Exhale on the brandish. Blow up! Inhale on stowing the blade.

Full credit for the name Pirate Princess goes to a patient of Ruth's, who decided this weird diagonal exercise needed an inspiring moniker.

Pulldown (Sitting or Standing Only)

Tie a knot in the resistance band and throw it to hang over the top of a door. Then close the door to keep the band in place. Hold band in front of you, a little above shoulder level. Hold wrists and elbows straight and pull the band to your body, outside of your hips into shoulder extension. Release. Repeat 5 to 20 reps.

Breathing: Exhale on the pulldown. Inhale on the release.

Rowing (Sitting or Standing Only)

Tie a knot in the resistance band and secure on the handle of a door that will latch afterward. Holding the band in front of you, pull your bent elbows back behind your body. Release. Repeat 5 to 20 times.

Breathing: Exhale on the row. Inhale on the release.

Progressions: Consider if this exercise challenges you differently in a wide stance or a split stance.

DUMBBELL EXERCISES

Dumbbells are used for resistance training. Use a weight that feels challenging to you, allows you to hold anatomical neutral in sitting and standing, and makes you feel slightly tired by 12 reps. Dumbbells are frequently found at yard sales. You can also use soup cans or shopping bags weighted with bags of rice, flour, some books, or anything available that gets you to your preferred weight. You can perform dumbbell exercises seated and standing. Starting with one arm at a time will challenge your ability to hold anatomical neutral from left to right and resist rotation, while both at the same time will challenge your ability to use your deep core and pressure management system. The goal is to keep the torso stable as you move the arms and learn to exercise without breath locking.

Biceps Curl

Hold a weight in each hand at your side. Get in anatomical neutral. Bend your elbow and pull the weight to your shoulder. Release. Repeat 5 to 12 times.

Breathing: Exhale on the curl. Blow up! Inhale on the release.

Forward Punch

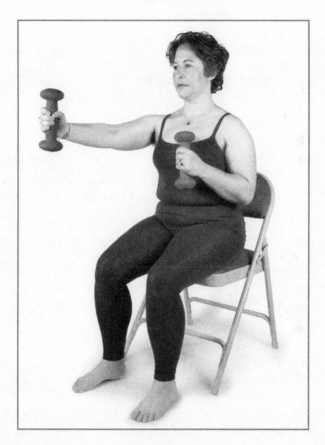

Get in anatomical neutral. Hold a weight in your hand like you are hold-ing a cup of coffee. Slowly push the weight forward until your elbow is straight. Do not allow your shoulder blade to reach, round, or push for-ward as the arm moves. Return to start. Repeat 5 to 12 times.

Breathing: Exhale on the punch. Inhale on the return.

CHAPTER 6

The Pelvic Floor

ANATOMY OF THE PELVIC FLOOR

The twenty or so pelvic floor muscles attach to the bottom of the pelvis along the pubis, ilia, ischia, sacrum, and coccyx. There is an anterior pelvic floor shaped like a triangle that we call the urogenital diaphragm. It supports the bladder and urethra and is most involved in urinary control, both holding in urine and allowing it to void fully. It also performs sexual health functions, holding the clitoris, secretory glands, and our vaginal/front opening.

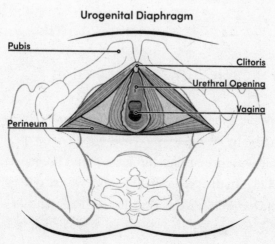

Urogenital Diaphragm

Pubis

Clitoris

Urethral Opening

Vagina

Perineum

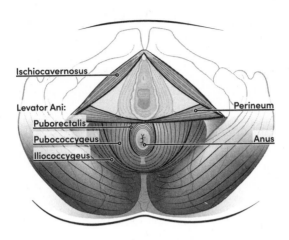

The deep or posterior pelvic floor helps control bowel function, pulling the rectum and sphincters up and forward to maintain control. The perineum is the muscle that delineates the anterior pelvic floor from the posterior pelvic floor, connecting the right and left sitz bones at the bottom of the ischia. Tension here helps both bowel and bladder function. Its position makes it always involved in the sexual function of the pelvic floor.

TENSING AND RELAXING

Pelvic Floor Muscle (PFM) Contraction

Tensing the pelvic floor, or the Kegel, is named after Dr. Arnold Kegel, a gynecologist who in 1948 published and popularized the idea that postpartum people with urinary incontinence could use muscle reeducation to reduce leaking. In the pelvic health world, we call a Kegel a *pelvic floor muscle contraction*. While Kegel's work is well-known and well cited, pelvic floor exercises were first described and published in 1936 by Margaret

Morris, a movement instructor, and Minnie Randell, a midwife, with rec-ommended use in the pregnant, postpartum, and postsurgical population to reduce incontinence. Despite the idea being around for over eighty years, research suggests that only 30 percent of people can contract their pelvic floors correctly. With training and education, that number goes up to 70 percent.

The only way you are going to see the action of the pelvic floor is na-ked in front of a mirror. Lying on your back with your knees bent, look at your genitals in a mirror and attempt to contract your pelvic floor. A con-traction should include the left, right, anterior, and posterior parts with a squeeze and lift. Visualizations can be helpful here. Imagine you are pull-ing your sitz bones together like elevator doors closing, closing your sphincters, holding in a fart, lifting your bladder up, or squeezing a tam-pon. You should see your anal sphincter contract and draw into the body, your perineum narrow and lift. As Morris and Randell describe it: "invert the sphincters . . . until it becomes habitual." Your vaginal/front opening should get smaller and lift into the body, and the clitoral hood and vulva will nod and flicker. Correctly tensing the pelvic floor involves two things: a squeeze and a lift, without any joints or bones moving, or the surrounding parts. Being able to isolate the pelvic floor will allow it to learn to contract no matter what the other parts of your body are doing. Practice holding the contraction for 3 to 5 seconds at first and then relax-ing fully. A common visualization is to imagine that you are stopping your urine stream (but please, please don't actually stop your urine stream).

The pelvic floor needs to function independently so that when other muscle groups are busy, it can work without their help. Customary cheats for Kegels are squeezing the buttocks, tilting the pelvis, squeezing the in-ner thighs, clenching the abs, holding your breath, or sucking in your breath with the Kegel or instead of it. Try to find the amount of effort that you can apply without any other muscles activating. Keep it light. If your muscles are weak, you might need to stick with breathing and visualiza-tion to start; trying harder will not generate a better outcome. This is just

Don't Stop the Streams: A Cautionary Tale

When Courtney was eleven years old, she happened upon her mother's copy of *Redbook* magazine in the bathroom. Did she leave it there so Courtney would read it? Who knows! It was full of many interesting and age-inappropriate things, so she read it avidly every month.

One issue had an article about Kegeling, probably in a "tight vagina = good sex" context, and it used the "stop the urine stream" example. Courtney tried it. And then every time she peed, she Kegeled.

Fast-forward two decades and change, to when Courtney was a new mother. She had a reputation for having to pee a lot, and it had only gotten worse postpartum. She and Ruth were hanging out at Ruth's house, and Courtney had to pee, so she went, and when she came out, Ruth was giving her a *look*.

"This is overstepping," she said, "but it sounds weird when you pee."

Excuse me?

"It sounds like you're stopping and starting a lot. Is that true?"

Courtney thought about it. She was in fact stopping and starting a lot. And having to push to get pee out. And then having to pee like two minutes later.

"Are you Kegeling while you pee?"

It turns out that Ruth is a bladder detective. Courtney's decades-long habit of pee-gel-ing had turned into dysfunction, and she and her hypertonic pelvic floor wound up in therapy. And that, dear readers, is why you should not stop the streams.

an isometric contraction, like making a fist. You're not squeezing lemons for lemonade. Make sure you can fully let go at the end and take a long break between each contraction to be sure you are not just getting tighter and tighter with time. What do we mean by that? It's possible that focusing on pelvic floor muscle contractions causes you to remain tight instead of relaxing. Contracting is great and useful, but it leads to problems if you don't relax between repetitions.

Graduated Positions for PFM Contractions

POSITION	DEGREE OF DIFFICULTY	DESCRIPTION
Gravity assisted	Easiest—you got this	Lying down, pelvis higher than the hips on a rolled blanket or pillow
Gravity neutral/ eliminated	Easy—typical exam posture	Side lying or lying on your back with knees bent
Against gravity	Medium challenging	Seated (easier when your legs are together, harder when they are apart)
Against gravity	Hard	Standing (difference in feet together vs. feet apart vs. one foot ahead of the other)
Dynamic against gravity	Expert level challenging	With lifting weight, standing on one leg, quick contraction with impact double leg, and then single leg

There's no right number of Kegels to do at a time or in a day. Everyone starts with different levels of fitness and muscle strength. If you birthed a baby, the method of delivery and degree of tearing will partly determine your areas of focus. Begin with a warmup and get yourself settled into the activity starting from an easy position. Contract and rest three times. Spend a few minutes focusing on the quality of the sensation of your Kegel and its coordination with your breathing, making sure you feel relaxation or a letdown movement on the inhale, and the upward movement or Kegel on the exhale. Blow up! Rather than counting your Kegels, which can change your focus from quality to quantity, stay present with your body. Stop when you no longer have the feeling of contracting or relaxing, or when you have tried and failed three times.

PFM Relaxation

Release the stranglehold! It might be counterintuitive, but Ruth sees plenty of folks asking to learn to do Kegels better when they actually have pelvic floor tension and need to learn to let go, not to tighten up. Relaxing is the absence of pressure and tension on the pelvic floor and surrounding fascia. The perineum will drop down like a bridge and be more visible in the mirror. The vaginal/front opening will be more visible and appear larger in width and length. The anal sphincter will be larger in width. The vulva will be soft. This should be accomplished without bearing down. Knowing how to do this is crucial for bladder and bowel emptying, having a strong urine stream, and being able to tolerate vaginal/front penetration. Coughing and sneezing are examples of times when the pelvic floor needs to let go and be at rest. In a healthy pelvic floor, the intra-abdominal pressure caused by forceful exhales should elicit a muscle co-contraction that is timed to keep you dry (exhale = diaphragm lifts, abs pull together and up, pelvic floor pulls together and up all in one go). This will not happen if you are already clenched. There is no natural responsiveness in a rigid system. It will respond paradoxically by giving out or bulging down, causing you to leak. This is where those 20,000 diaphragm breaths a day come in handy. If you've mastered your inhale down, the pelvic floor has been lightly stretched with every inhale and learned to recoil on your exhales.

Again, visualizations are helpful. Imagine the opening of the vagina/front hole is like a tightly closed flower. Inhale and pull your breath down to that flower. Imagine the flower blooming and opening. Picture the perineum dropping down like a bridge. Sit on a washcloth and feel the pelvic floor expanding down into the washcloth. (The most it really moves is 1 to 2 centimeters.) Sitting on exercise balls and foam rollers enhances the feeling of pelvic floor lengthening and relaxation. Remember, this is just as important as learning how to tighten.

We recommend trying the "let go" part of the Kegel in the same positions we listed above, from easiest to hardest. Give yourself feedback by squeezing gently and then releasing, which builds confidence in knowing the difference between tensing and relaxing. Rethink traditional Kegel training by doubling the amount of time you spend in the resting phase. For example, if you contract and hold a Kegel for 5 seconds, then spend at least 10 seconds in relaxation.

Some folks develop clenching behaviors due to leakage or prolapse symptoms (heaviness, pressure, falling out feeling, or a bulge that you can see or feel). It makes sense that when we believe things are leaking or loose that they need to be tightened, but your perception of your pelvic floor may not equal reality. Giving birth does not mean stretched-out genitals or pelvic floor. Without being evaluated by a professional, like a PT or OT skilled in pelvic health, or your ob-gyn or midwife, you just don't know your pelvic floor situation. This means that leaning into Kegels—long holds, multiple repetitions, multiple sets, 100 Kegels a day, or Kegeling at every stoplight—is not the answer. Coordination of the pelvic floor in re- lationship to the other body systems it communicates with is the answer. That cannot be achieved if our only relationship with our pelvic floor in- volves clenching it all the time.

Another reason the pelvic floor can be tense is habit. This comes from following cues to suck in your belly, pull your belly button into your spine, or flatten your back to the mat, often heard in fitness classes. Some classes even recommend adding a Kegel or belly-flattening maneuver to move- ments when that contraction wouldn't naturally occur. Our bodies are smart. They will do what they have always done to save energy. It will take attention to realize this is your habit before you can change it. Allow yourself to let go of the pelvic floor and fully relax your abdominal mus- cles, even if you worry that you will pee or your organs will fall out (they won't). This idea is born out of fear and body shame. You don't need that to feel better, and tension as a response may cause the outcome you fear.

Alternatively, the pelvic floor can be tight due to stress, fear, or panic. In this context our symptomatic pelvic floors may be asking for TLC, just like our tight shoulders and backs let us know we need care and attention. A tense pelvic floor can cause overactive bladder (peeing a lot), leakage with cough/laugh/sneeze, bladder pain with filling or emptying, a feeling that you can't empty completely or have a weird urine stream, an inability to tolerate sex, constipation, a sensation that your bowels won't empty even when they feel full, pain with pooping, and pain in the pelvis, hip, or spine that doesn't go away with usual strategies or treatments. This tension is a maladaptive protective response. You are trying to keep your body safe. This can be due to a traumatic birth, a difficult postpartum transition, pain, overexertion, a triggered emotional response from birth, and re-traumatization caused by birth. In this context, you need to check in with yourself. The contract/relax is a great way to gauge your tension. Breathing is essential to calming the nervous system, so master the exercises in chapter 4 before seeking out Kegels. Journaling your feelings about birth, your body, your relationship, your new role as parent, or infant loss can help, too.

Prompts

1. What about your birth makes you want to clench?
2. Is there anything in your experience with your body that taught you that tighter is better? Is that still serving you?
3. How might you feel unsafe with your body as it is right now?
4. What activities make your muscles and body feel soft, pliable, and responsive? How can you fit those into your current lifestyle?
5. Can you accept that a pliable pelvic floor is more responsive to your needs and will reduce your symptoms? If so, what can you do to foster that? If not, why not?

THE PRESSURE MANAGEMENT SYSTEM

The function of the pelvic floor is to react and respond to your environment in order to support your internal organs and sphincter closure without your having to think about it. By the time a person has mastered walking and is potty-trained—usually around three or four years old—the pelvic floor has developed enough to support basic body movements and to keep urine and stool on the inside. We do not, and should not, teach three-year-olds how to Kegel. Instead, we teach them to pay attention to their body sensations and to use the bathroom at regular intervals until they learn to remain continent in the daytime. These kiddos can run, jump, climb, cough, and sneeze all over everyone without peeing their pants (most of the time) because their pelvic floor, organ, and sphincter supports are integrated into their regular body movements. They unconsciously absorb and respond to impact with a squeeze and a lift. That's the goal for the postpartum pelvic floor, too. You can get back there. You can. Give it time.

The way into the pressure management system is to coordinate breath with pelvic floor tension and relaxation. You already know breath-holding is a strategy for building stability. But that strategy can cause a weak and healing pelvic floor to bulge. When the pelvic floor bulges, it doesn't do its job well, which results in leakage, prolapse, or pain. This is the primary reason *not* to Kegel by sucking in. If you can't Kegel on an exhale, then you might leak on one instead.

Your pelvic floor is the literal foundation of the pressure management system. Strengthening the muscles above your pelvic floor before you can Kegel and relax on demand can increase downward pressure, resulting in more weakness and difficulty contracting when your pelvic floor needs to work. The goal is coordination of the entire pressure management system, or deep core, which includes the pelvic floor, diaphragm, abs, and spinal muscles.

SEXUAL HEALTH

Returning to pleasurable and enjoyable sexual function is one of the most empowering and frustrating parts of postpartum recovery. Connecting intimately can restore a bond with a partner, but it can also cause a relationship divide when your body functions differently from how it used to. Many folks get the all clear at their six-week visit but quickly find out that they weren't ready to return to intimacy. It's common to feel fearful in the face of knowing when and if it's the right time to try again, which can lead to avoidance. Some may self-medicate to try to "get through it" (which is never recommended). Postpartum couples describe levels of reduced satisfaction, reduced desire, and increased sexual distress. Yes, couples! The non-birthing partner may be worried about your health and happiness and may suffer similar sleepless nights, limiting parasympathetic nervous system function. This is not a condemnation of the changes in your body size and shape. This is also not a reason to be doing 100 Kegels or trying to Kegel during sex. We want you to understand your postpartum body better to reduce this pain, shame, and blame cycle.

There are a few benchmark questions to answer before returning to sexual activity. First, are your tissues healed enough to be touched? Has your delivery team verified that your scars, including from cesarean birth, are closed, mobile, and able to tolerate touch? Is your risk for injury and infection low? Have you established your birth control priorities? If you are not using birth control, would you feel okay if a pregnancy occurred from being sexually active? This is a fertile time, and typical methods of non-medicated birth control may not be reliable. Make sure that you are physically prepared and your provider doesn't anticipate any adverse outcomes. Ask them these questions if you aren't sure—they've heard it all before.

Returning to sexual function requires you to know your own values and desires. How would you like to show up in your sexual life? How do you prioritize your sexuality? What parts of your sexual experience make you feel most engaged? How ready are you to experience touch? Are there places on your body that you do not want your partner to touch? How much bandwidth do you have to give in a sexual capacity? Are there intimacy needs that make you feel more fulfilled? Do you need to orgasm? Are you okay with engaging in non-penetrative intimacy? Do you need some form of penetrative intimacy? Is it better if you see your partner face-to-face? Do you prefer to spend a certain amount of time with your partner before initiating penetration?

Female and Assigned Female at Birth Sexual Function

Sexual function for females and those assigned female at birth (AFAB) is typically measured in six domains: desire, arousal, lubrication, orgasm, satisfaction, and the presence of any pain.

- ☐ **Desire:** Do you have an intrinsic interest in sexual activity? Are you able to respond to a partner's desire? Are there activities/fantasies that increase your sexual desire? Are there activities or circumstances that reduce your desire?

- ☐ **Arousal:** Are you able to engage in stimulating activities or fantasies that cause adequate genital engorgement, vaginal/genital opening, stiffening, and lengthening? Do you wait to start penetrative activities until you are fully aroused? Do you give yourself enough time to try to become fully aroused?

- ☐ **Lubrication:** Do your body's glands and tissues create and sustain their own lubrication to the start and completion of your sexual activity? Do you own a lubricant that you can use and have nearby in case your body is not producing enough lubrication? Is that lubrication compatible with the condoms or toys you use?

☐ **Orgasm:** Are you able to achieve one? How difficult is it to attain? Do you prefer to continue sexual activity until you achieve an orgasm? Are there areas of your body that help you have one more readily?

☐ **Satisfaction:** Are you connecting with your partner during sexual activity in a way that feels fulfilling and supportive (or yourself if engaging in autoerotic activities)?

☐ **Pain:** Is any act of penetration or sexual stimulation uncomfortable? Do you stop or modify your activities when this pain occurs? Are there ways to be sexually active and stay away from your painful areas?

Do you know the answers to these questions? If not, spend some time really thinking about the things you need to hash out and clarify. Some of them are better answered after a bout of self-stimulation. Many people feel this is wasteful or selfish. It is not selfish to know your body and its responses better. It is not wasteful to spend time figuring out what touch is comfortable and what touch is painful before you expect a partner to do that for you. No one knows your body better than you. Your finding out what works is investigative and will be instructive to a partner when you do have the time and energy to be together again.

Two key elements for successful encounters are arousal and lubrication. Arousal sets the stage for penetration tolerance and orgasm. Without it, pain will be higher and satisfaction lower. Arousal can even drive desire. In females and AFABs, desire may not occur until you are already aroused. Lubrication makes the difference between tolerance or intolerance of friction and repetitive touch. Again, without it, pain will be higher, satisfaction lower, and it can be difficult to achieve orgasm (even with external stimulation only). Breastfeeding, chestfeeding, and lactating change your sex hormone production and reduce the hormones that stimulate vaginal/genital secretions. You can be fully aroused and still feel dry. Therefore, having a lubricant that is safe and effective is paramount. Do not measure your level of arousal by the amount of self-lubrication that occurs.

Lubrication

Unfortunately, many lubricants have additives and chemical formulas that are irritating to your sensitive genital tissue. If it stings, doesn't last, makes you sore or itchy, or leaves a strange residue, then it's not working for you. Read the labels and steer clear of these additives:

- Propylene glycol
- Glycerin
- Parabens
- Chlorhexidine gluconate
- Petrolatum
- Artificial flavorings
- Warming agents

Finding the Right Lubricant for Your Needs

TYPE OF LUBE	CONDOMS?	I USE TOYS . . .	THINGS TO CONSIDER . . .	BRANDS
Water-based	Compatible	Compatible	• Not very viscous. • Easily absorbed or evaporated. • May need reapplication. • Best for folks with sensitive skin.	• Sliquid H$_2$O • Slippery Stuff • Blossom Organics • Sutil
Silicone-based	Likely compatible	Not for silicone-based toys. Compatible for others.	• Can be too lubricating, resulting in reduced sensation. • Most recommended for birth scars and injuries. • Reduces friction-based pain. • Best for comfort with skin-to-skin contact.	• Überlube • Pink

Finding the Right Lubricant for Your Needs

TYPE OF LUBE	CONDOMS?	I USE TOYS ...	THINGS TO CONSIDER ...	BRANDS
Aloe-based (water-based)	Compatible	Compatible	• Can absorb or evaporate quickly. Can dry sticky with a residue. • Great for sore/red/ inflamed skin. More viscous than water-based.	• Good Clean Love • Desert Harvest
Oils	Not compatible! Breakage alert!	Compatible	• Oil can stain textiles/products. • Not always enough to create a slick effect to reduce friction/scar tissue pain.	• Standard store-bought coconut oil, almond oil, sunflower oil, or grape-seed oil • Vmagic

Resumption of Sexual Activity

When returning to partnered sexual activity, communication is key. Speak about your expectations. Unmet and unspoken expectations can lead to resentment. Work together to create an environment that's conducive to relaxation and intimacy, using whatever techniques get you going—aromatherapy, mood lighting, massage, bathing, music, or uninterrupted time together. Arousal lives in the part of your nervous system that is relaxed, well fed, and well cared for, the parasympathetic nervous system. Address any elements that might be getting in the way: an unlocked door, a dirty room, household chores that need attending, the determination of who is getting up for the nightly feeding. Speak with your partner about what needs could be taken off your plate to give you more energy to apply to your relationship. Involve them in the planning process to enhance foreplay in the forms of anticipation and desire. Shop for toys and tools to prioritize your sensory needs for arousal, orgasm, and fulfillment, such as a vibrator, a penis sleeve, or a cock ring.

Prioritize connection, intimacy, and pleasure through non-penetrative intercourse without the specter of pain with penetration clouding your experience. Hold yourself and your partner accountable for maintaining any boundaries you've set. This conversation is most productive outside of the bedroom when no one's immediate sexual fulfillment is on the line. Give your genitals positive experiences to improve later interest and desire, and progress to penetrative encounters when you know your needs for arousal, lubrication, and lack of pain are met. View every encounter as novel. What happened last time won't necessarily happen this time, for better or worse. Be true to what enhances the connection and pleasure you have with your partner.

Pain with Intercourse

How to resolve pain during sexual encounters? Start with nonverbal hand-over-hand guidance. Say, "Try this," to suggest something that might feel better, and remember that *no* and *stop* are always available. Ask explicitly for more of something that is working for you. Give your partner avenues to continue in an intimate and supportive way. Use more lubricant. Change positions. Stop penetration but continue external stimulation if that's comfortable. Say no, firmly but clearly, if you experience pain or reach a point where you need all activity to end. This will reduce strife in your relationship and protect you from further harm. Continuing acts of intimacy that are painful because you don't want to say no may result in more pain next time. Saying yes when you mean no can cause relational harm to both of you, but honest communication can build trust, connection, and intimacy. A number of specific conditions can lead to pain with intercourse, including:

VAGINAL/GENITAL BIRTH TEARS OR EPISIOTOMIES

Vaginal/genital birth tears and episiotomies are skin disruptions that need to heal before your return to intercourse. They should be free of signs of inflammation: redness, swelling, pain, and heat. Coconut oil (or the alternatives in the chart above) applied nightly can reduce sensitivity to touch and give you the opportunity to slowly touch, stretch, and move your scars. It also hydrates the tissue to enhance healing and pliability.

Pain with intercourse after tearing or scarring is often described as a raw or dry feeling, like sandpaper or a speed bump. You may be able to tolerate vaginal/front penetration but have sensitivity to friction. If you can tolerate penetrative intercourse, use the most pain-free positions, outlined later in this chapter. Communicate with your partner to let them know which areas to avoid touching and use a lot of lubricant. Commit to non-penetrative intimacy if your friction tolerance is low. Use a pelvic wand 1 to 10 minutes two to four days a week with gentle pressure to improve the mobility of the perineum and the scar's ability to stretch. The perineum must be able to move downward to allow for comfortable penetration.

VAGINISMUS

Vaginismus is a reflexive spasm of the first layer of the pelvic floor at the vaginal/front opening. The right and left sides come together so tightly that it is painful or impossible to separate them beyond the introitus or vaginal/front opening. This can happen following a vaginal/genital or cesarean birth.

Vaginismus is more common in people with a history of sexual assault or trauma, because for some, the sensation of a vaginal/genital delivery or sensations related to an episiotomy or tearing bring back similar sensations.

Your pelvic floor and other muscles respond to pain with panic, fear, and protective tension. They can be tight all the time, or only in response to penetration attempts. Unsuccessful or painful intercourse, often in the name of "taking one for the team," can lead to secondary trauma. You

Postpartum Humans:
AMY G.

PROBLEM

Amy found that after her vaginal delivery with tearing, she was unable to have pain-free penetrative intercourse with her partner. Her partner was someone she trusted, had established a good relationship with, and had had pleasurable and pain-free intercourse with prior to birth. The novel sensation of pain after birth was so like what she experienced during an assault that it took her aback. She was not prescreened for trauma by any member of her medical team and was unprepared for this possibility, despite having undergone extensive therapy for her assault many years prior. She thought she was "done with it." She had done the work to heal. She had a great relationship with her spouse. She didn't think this terrible old experience would show up in childbirth. Yet here she was, unable to relax or tolerate penetrative sex.

SOLUTION

Amy started pelvic floor PT, worked through visualization for birth trauma, and read *Mothering from Your Center* by Tami Lynn Kent at the recommendation of her therapist. This conversation was a catalyst to realizing what was happening with her was not just a "tissue issue" and had a deeper emotional basis. Amy found a technique for trauma healing called Brainspotting, developed by David Grand, PhD, which provided significant relief. This technique is an offshoot of EMDR and uses fixed eye positions to treat trauma. She knew that her amygdala and hippocampus were conspiring against her and bringing her back to her assault based on the sensations her body was experiencing.

Amy combined mental health treatment with pelvic floor PT to return to intercourse without pain, after using a pelvic wand to work on her scar tissue touch and mobility tolerance. When she was ready to restart penetration, she used plenty of lube, and her partner communicated so well and was so worried about hurting her, she had to tell him to shut up because he was ruining the mood!

may feel broken or believe that you can never have pleasurable intercourse again. It isn't true. Your amygdala, that reactive cave-person midbrain, is perpetuating a cycle of fear. We call this your internal heckler. The heckler misinterprets situations similar to the ones that caused prior pain or your fear of experiencing pain and turns them into hypersensitivity, tension, and hypervigilance. The heckler will keep you from getting "in the mood," aroused, or even attempting to engage in any acts of intimacy. The tension created from these limiting sensations can prove it correct when things are uncomfortable or painful and start the cycle anew.

How can you break that cycle? Feed your brain's internal cheerleader and starve that heckler! Embrace pleasurable touch. Focus on non-penetrative arousal, satisfaction, and orgasm. With your partner, agree to no penetration, no matter how good foreplay feels in the moment, until you are sure that your pelvic floor is pain-free to touch, stretching, and dilating by other means. Sign a written contract if that helps you stick to the plan.

Using a dilator or pelvic wand gradually increases the tolerance to length and girth of your tissues. They train your muscles and your brain not to overreact to the sensations of penetration, stretch, and friction. Start slow and skinny, with just a finger, and always use plenty of lubrication. Insert a small dilator or wand for 1 to 10 minutes two to four days a week. Increase the size and movement of the device when the smallest size is easy to insert without pain. You should be able to use the device to push into the left, right, and posterior parts of the pelvic floor before progressing to a larger size. A sex-literate social worker, sex therapist, and/or pelvic health therapist can provide help and guidance.

DYSPAREUNIA

Painful intercourse without an apparent muscle spasm is called dyspareunia. This can be the result of vaginal/genital dryness or friction on the tissues as they heal. The basic recommendations are the same: Check for healing and signs of inflammation, use coconut oil (or another recommended oil) every night, and make sure you can tolerate self-touch on well-lubricated healing tissues. Try dilators or a pelvic wand to help get your tissues ready for penetration. Using a device-compatible lubricant is key, as is remembering to reapply water-based lubricants if you feel any dryness, scratchiness, or pulling with movement.

POSITIONAL PAIN WITH INTERCOURSE

Some pain with intercourse occurs due to musculoskeletal or pelvic pain after pregnancy and delivery. This can mean the pain is not genital in origin but may become genital pain if your pelvic floor decides to protect you—i.e., spasm and create tension—or your cesarean birth scar is not fully pliable, blocking you from having comfortable sex.

The position of your body, including your spine and legs, can make a huge difference. Consider trying the position(s) from this table that meet your needs and see what changes.

Penetrative Positioning Options

POSITION	BENEFITS	EFFECTS POST-CESAREAN BIRTH	CONSIDERATIONS
Side-lying	• Limits depth of penetration • Keeping legs together reduces hip and pubis pain • Reduced thrusting for back pain • No pressure on labia	• No pressure on the scar • No need to hold the legs or use the core • No pain from scar friction	• Use the Ohnut or a similar product to limit depth of penetration • Not face-to-face • The top side will have more vaginal/genital and labial friction (if you tore keep this in mind) • Will need supplemental clitoral stimulation
You on top	• Increased autonomy • Face-to-face • More control over depth, thrust	• No pressure on the scar • Requires some core activation	• Very athletic—may not be able to continue for a long time due to fatigue • Can be done on knees or on feet • Increased labial rub/pressure/friction if leg control is poor

Penetrative Positioning Options

POSITION	BENEFITS	EFFECTS POST-CESAREAN BIRTH	CONSIDERATIONS
You on your back	• Face-to-face • Access to clitoral stimulation • You will do less of the work	• Heavy on the core (holding legs in the air) • Increased touch to scar	• May require Ohnut to limit depth of penetration • Less control over depth and rate • Increased friction to labia/perineal tear • May aggravate pubis or SI joint pain • Use wedge pillow under hips to reduce angle on introitus
Hands and knees	• Reduces leg and spine work • Access to clitoral stimulation	• No pressure on scar • Belly hanging down may be relaxing or aggravating	• May require Ohnut to reduce depth of penetration • No face-to-face • Can lean over something to brace spine • Less labial pressure

CONDITIONS OF PELVIC FLOOR DYSFUNCTION

Constipation

Get ready to talk about poop! Constipation is arguably the most serious pelvic floor dysfunction. If you have constipation, you can have a host of related issues, like prolapse, urinary incontinence, urinary urgency, urinary frequency, and pain. Constipation is defined as infrequent or irregular bowel movements, fewer than three per week, *and* difficulty with letdown during a bowel movement, painful bowel movements, a feeling of incomplete emptying, or a persistent feeling of heaviness, bloating, or gas after eating.

The good news is that you can resolve constipation with lifestyle changes, meaning rest, hydration, and nutrition. Sound familiar? Those 48 ounces of water, 28 grams of fiber, adequate sleep, and regularity with eating are necessary for consistent bowel movements. Your parasympathetic nervous system is the "rest and digest" portion of your central nervous system, so if you're stressed and spending all your time in "fight or flight," your digestion and excretion will be negatively impacted. Before you consider taking any supplements or other interventions for your bowels, make sure you're meeting the basics.

Practice healthy bowel habits. Poop within 30 minutes of feeling the urge. Sit all the way down on the toilet with your knees higher than your hips. Use a stool if you are short (or your toilet is too high). Don't bear down! That is like forcing your pelvic floor to "give birth" every time you poop. Aren't you trying to recover from the birthing process? Bearing down more, for any reason, is going to limit your goal achievement. It reduces your pelvic floor strength and increases your risk of urinary incontinence, hemorrhoids, and pelvic organ prolapse. If you're having difficulty getting the poop out, wait a bit, go for a walk, drink some water, gently rub your belly, dance (or do some other relaxed movement), and then go back to the toilet when you feel the urge return. Sometimes people need a distraction because they are *too* into their poo. Limit your toilet sitting to no more than 3 to 5 minutes at a time. Vocalizations can assist in bowel production without pelvic floor injury, much as they are used in birth. Humming, saying *mooooo*, or creating a raspberry sound with your lips while sitting on the toilet encourages your pelvic floor to relax. Yes, we know that's weird. This whole section probably feels a little weird. We're in it together.

Constipation can be caused by pelvic floor tension. Try holding the perineum up with your fingers when you need to poop and it won't come out. This is called splinting. You can also try a wand called the Femmeze or the CMT Release device, which holds the perineum for you. This allows the internal and external anal sphincters to relax.

If you are still unable to pass a full BM, have added fiber and water to your diet, have support under your feet so that your knees are higher than hips, and have actively worked to relax on the toilet to no avail, use a vibrator on the perineum externally up to 10 minutes a few days a week to improve blood flow and reduce tension. Work on breathing into the perineum and practicing pelvic floor relaxation rather than Kegel training. Some pelvic health therapists also treat constipation if you are not seeing improvements.

If you're still having issues, talk to your provider about supplements, laxatives, or stool softeners that might be safe for you. This could include magnesium glycinate or magnesium citrate; stool softeners like docusate sodium (common brand: Colace); glycerin suppositories, or laxatives like polyethylene glycol. Stimulant laxatives, supplements, or teas like senna can be habit-forming and can cause dependence, constipation, and pain with long-term use. Find out what your provider recommends and go from there.

Urinary Incontinence

Urinary incontinence, or involuntary loss of urine, is the reason Margaret Morris, Minnie Randell, and Dr. Arnold Kegel advanced the idea of pelvic floor strengthening in the first place. Urinary incontinence has multiple causes and types of presentation, and each type of leakage has different solutions. Take note, Kegels are not one size fits all.

URGE INCONTINENCE
Urge incontinence occurs shortly after feeling like it's time to pee. Urgency can be caused by low water intake/dehydration, increased irritant intake, constipation, or fear of leakage. A tight pelvic floor can put pressure on the urethra, causing irritation and a constant sense of needing to

go, even if there isn't much fluid volume. Increase your fluid intake and follow the urge control protocol.

Urge Control Protocol

1. **Stop!** DO NOT RUN TO THE BATHROOM. You will never outrun your bladder. Get still and do not give in to panic.
2. **Breathe.** Get your nervous system calmed down and under control. Having a full bladder is not an emergency. Breathing deeply and slowly convinces your system that you are safe.
3. **Think positive thoughts.** Try "I can make it" or "I am no more full now than I was two minutes ago." Alternatively, distract yourself by singing a song or thinking about something else.
4. **Try Kegels.** Rhythmically squeeze, lift, and then release your pelvic floor. If you lean forward slightly, this aims the contraction at your bladder rather than at your anus. This also tells the bladder to knock it off, stop being dramatic about being full, and get back to its number one job, holding your urine in.

Repeat as often as needed to calmly and confidently walk to the bathroom, or before your common triggers.

Types of Urinary Incontinence and Treatment Approaches

TYPE OF INCONTINENCE	SYMPTOMS	WHAT ARE SOME POTENTIAL SOLUTIONS?	WHEN SHOULD I SEE A PROFESSIONAL?
Urge incontinence	• Urgent need to pee • Feeling like you won't make it on time • Frequent urination	• Hydrate • Reduce bladder irritants • Reduce just-in-case or high-frequency toileting • Employ urge control protocol • Reduce PFM tension • Manage constipation	• Unable to resolve with lifestyle changes • Unable to perform household or work functions due to frequency

Types of Urinary Incontinence and Treatment Approaches

TYPE OF INCONTINENCE	SYMPTOMS	WHAT ARE SOME POTENTIAL SOLUTIONS?	WHEN SHOULD I SEE A PROFESSIONAL?
Stress incontinence	● Leakage with activity: · Cough · Laugh · Sneeze · Lift · Yell · Run · Jump	● The Knack (page 156) ● Piston breathing with exercise (page 225) ● Kegels with great form ● Stop ALL straining ● Strengthen surrounding muscle groups	● Leakage that you cannot control ● Inability to do daily tasks without leaking
Nocturia	● Getting up to pee more than once a night ● Urination that regularly interrupts restful sleep	● Eliminate daytime just-in-case peeing ● Stay hydrated during the day ● Reduce bladder irritants ● Stop drinking two hours before bedtime ● Try urge control protocol and go back to sleep	● Getting up three or more times at night
Overactive bladder	● Peeing frequently with poor output ● Not able to hold the bladder more than two hours	● Stress management, mindfulness, or relaxation 10 to 20 minutes daily ● Reduction of irritants ● Urge control protocol ● Manage constipation ● Reduce PFM tension	● Frequent inability to hold it more than two hours during the day ● Constant symptoms of urge regardless of when you last emptied ● Recurrent UTI
Mixed incontinence	● Leaking with urge, stress, and triggers of movement or environment	● All of the above recommendations apply	● Symptoms not managed with lifestyle changes or exercise ● Constant drip feeling without control

STRESS URINARY INCONTINENCE (SUI)

Stress urinary incontinence is leakage associated with a physical trigger or stressor. Common stressors are coughing, laughing, sneezing, lifting, changing position, running, and jumping. Using a well-executed Kegel before or with your triggers can keep you dry. This is called the Knack, as in timing is everything. Train yourself to Kegel before or with forceful exhalations like a cough/laugh/sneeze. This works in the short term. In

---

Postpartum Humans: HM

PROBLEM

Prior to pregnancy, HM experienced mild stress incontinence. She had seen a pelvic floor physical therapist for pain during her third trimester. Her delivery was difficult. She had a catheter inserted during labor that was removed too quickly during a vacuum-assisted vaginal delivery with episiotomy. While still in the hospital, she began to experience severe loss of bladder control every time she moved from sitting to standing. She had to frequently rush to the bathroom, soaking through pads, and found she was able to walk for only a few seconds before losing control. She received inconsistent suggestions from her providers; lying in the hospital bed at two days postpartum, she was told she would likely have incontinence for the rest of her life. She was given recommendations ranging from a book and a feedback device to assurances that the condition would resolve quickly on its own. She left the hospital feeling hopeless and without support. When she attended a postpartum appointment for her child in a wheelchair due to the severity of her symptoms, a passing midwife spotted her and immediately wrote a referral to pelvic floor physical therapy.

SOLUTION

After only two visits to the pelvic floor physical therapist, HM's most severe symptoms were corrected. Knowing how to perform a good Kegel was the first step in her return to higher-level activities like hiking, going for walks, running, and yoga.

the long term, restoring the normal mechanics of the diaphragm so that it lifts with the rest of the deep core (abdominals, pelvic floor, and spinal muscles) is the real answer. Jumping, running, and changing position require your pelvic floor to function as a trampoline, absorbing and responding to impact, as covered in chapter 10. With enough training, the pelvic floor will return to lifting and contracting reflexively. Stay out of your own way by not holding tension all the time and eliminating bearing down, which trains the pelvic floor to give out under pressure.

HM's story illustrates stress incontinence at its most severe and demonstrates the importance of pelvic floor strengthening. Your pelvic floor needs to have enough resting muscle tone so you can stand without peeing. Kegels are the way to achieve that low-level control, but do not automatically translate to the dynamic control needed for sports.

MIXED INCONTINENCE

Mixed incontinence has elements of both urge incontinence and stress incontinence. Ruth sees a lot of patients who begin with stress incontinence— a leak with a cough, laugh, or sneeze. This leads people to drink less water and do a lot of just-in-case toileting, signaling their brain that "urine is bad." This leads to a lower tolerance for bladder filling and more concentrated urine.

Dehydration, constipation, and bladder irritation will result in having to go all the time, but not having a lot of volume when you do. This restricts the bladder from being able to expand and opens the door to bearing down to empty the bowels. These secondary circumstances, mostly self-inflicted, have now caused urge incontinence. All this adds up to mixed urinary incontinence. Fix water intake issues by increasing slowly over the day until you are comfortably back at 48 ounces minimum. Convince yourself that needing to pee is not the enemy. Eliminate just-in-case toileting by trusting your bladder when you can. Practice exercises for reintegrating your pelvic floor with your pressure management system.

Practice the Knack for predictable symptoms of leakage. Train with the exercises at the end of chapter 7 for hip and core integration.

Pelvic Organ Prolapse

Pelvic organ prolapse refers to a descent of any of the pelvic organs from their normal anatomical positions. This creates a sensation of something "falling out," heaviness, pressure, or back pain and can lead to incomplete emptying of the bladder and/or bowel, including difficulty initiating emptying. Pelvic organ prolapse occurs most frequently in postpartum people who had a vaginal/genital delivery, tearing, forceps or vacuum-assisted delivery, and/or an episiotomy. The bigger the tear or episiotomy, the more likely it is that you will have a pelvic organ prolapse in your lifetime.

Each type of pelvic organ prolapse is similar in presentation, with a sensation of heaviness, of something you can see and/or feel in the vagina/genitals that wasn't there before. A cystocele or rectocele looks like a balloon in the vaginal/front opening. A uterine prolapse causes the cervix to present lower down in the vagina so that a person can feel it with their finger—it typically feels like the tip of your nose. A prolapsed urethra looks like a striped tube. A vaginal/genital prolapse presents with the sensation that "things" are more in the way than they used to be and can produce *vaginal wind,* also known as a queef. Vaginal wind is an involuntary passage of odorless air through the vagina/front hole, which is often audible and/or sensible and usually associated with a change in posture. This may occur when the legs are abducted and a change of position occurs, and during times of low estrogen (e.g., lactating).

Getting evaluated by a gynecologist allows you to understand your options for medical treatment. If you suspect a prolapse because you're feeling the sensations we've described, see your doctor. Prolapse is non-life-threatening and treatable, and as with all medical decisions, there are pros and cons to every approach based on your history and circumstances.

Because most people aren't aware that prolapse after birth is a possibility, suspecting you have one can feel overwhelming and scary. Don't panic, and don't blame yourself! Prolapses just happen, regardless of your level of strength and fitness. Here is a list of things you can do to reduce the impact of your prolapse, both before your first medical appointment and after any surgical interventions.

1. Create and maintain a good bowel routine that does not cause you to sit on the toilet too long or strain.

2. If you have symptoms of incomplete emptying, use the splint for bowel emptying or hold your lower belly up with your hands for bladder emptying. This reduces the urge to strain. Standing up and sitting right back down to empty a second time can get those last drips out.

3. Work on finding your Kegel. Use a mirror to see if your Kegel reduces your prolapse (that's the goal). It should shrink in size and be drawn into the body.

4. Do breathing exercises every day that allow you to fully relax and be more aware of your muscle tension.

5. Spend 10 to 20 minutes in the evening getting gravity and your body weight off your pelvis. Try legs up on a therapy ball or legs up the wall. These positions pair well with breathing and Kegels.

6. Pay attention to activities that consistently make you more symptomatic, where the pelvic floor should add support but isn't able to do so effectively, like lifting, bending, pushing, pulling, or carrying. Modify or reduce these activities when you can. It's not realistic to avoid them altogether, but practicing smaller or less frequent load management will help you get better at larger and more frequent tasks.

7. Get really good at the activities in this chapter and Piston breathing (chapter 10) to improve your coordination.

8. Do not google it. Just don't. You will encounter horror stories and see photos you can't unsee. Fear is not what you want to cultivate here.

9. Go for regular walks. Start small and try not to wear an infant or push a stroller if possible. Start with 10 minutes three to five days a week and keep the intensity low. Build slowly over time as you feel the prolapse less or recover more quickly. Walking on an incline is more difficult but can improve your posture and help fire other supportive muscles, like the gluteals.

10. If an activity makes you symptomatic, get off your pelvis, breathe, Kegel, and be kind to your body. Do whatever you can to keep from catastrophizing. Symptoms of prolapse can be worse when you are stressed.

11. It's okay to have sex with a prolapse. Your partner may not notice anything is different at all. Use a lubricant, find positions that make your prolapse feel less prominent, and don't bear down into an orgasm. If you are worried about organ symptoms like heaviness, pressure, or possibly incontinence, do a gentle bowel cleanout, or urinate just prior.

Most people have more prolapse symptoms while standing. This might lead you to believe that you should stand less. This is another maladaptive pattern people employ to try to resolve their symptoms. It will backfire. Standing less or exercising only on your back will reduce your tolerance for standing. Exercise works with prolapse management by encouraging blood flow, breath coordination, and general tone. Exercise that trains you bottom up, like stairs or step-ups, can assist the pelvic floor in supporting the organs. What might need to be avoided is too much abdominal work. Increasing pressure on the abdominal cavity (which occurs in most programs that involve lying on your back) and employing the "belly button to spine" cue will increase intra-abdominal pressure and can send your organs down if you haven't mastered your diaphragm/abs/pelvic floor coordination exercises yet.

Prolapse is going to tattle on you even more than pelvic floor tension will; that is to say, you will experience more symptoms of prolapse when you are not getting your basic needs met. Rest, hydration, nutrition, and exercise are the recipe to living in harmony with a prolapse. In fact, because prolapse is associated with tissue weakness and muscle endurance, you may need to eat *more* protein and fiber to keep yourself feeling well. Your prolapse might act up with too much rest or too much exercise. It's a mind game, for sure. Settle in for the long haul. There might be days that you are symptomatic for no good reason. There might be days you are symptomatic, and you damn well know the reason and can't do anything about it. When you can, do something that you know helps you feel better. On days when you're feeling brave, try a little extra. You might surprise yourself.

If you can't stand the sensation and symptoms of prolapse, talk to your ob-gyn about a pessary fitting, topical medications for muscle bulking, or surgery. A pessary is a disc inserted deep into the vagina that acts like a brace for the organs. Pessaries come in many shapes and sizes and are typically made of medical-grade silicone; many can be removed by you or your partner. Wearing a pessary for prolapse is like wearing an ankle brace for an ankle sprain: your body is not suddenly perfect, but it allows you to stay in the game. For some, it improves strengthening of the pelvic floor and core.

Some prolapses require surgery. There is a failure rate to surgery, and it's typically associated with "re-prolapsing." This could happen if you lost the genetic lottery for tissue integrity, but is more likely to occur if you don't change the habits that contribute to prolapse. These include pushing, straining, holding your breath, strenuous bearing down, or con-

tinuously building abdominal pressure in every exercise. If you have constipation, get that shit under control. If you are a chronic exerciser, work on integration exercises, rather than pushing hard 100 percent of the time.

PELVIC FLOOR MUSCLE EXERCISES

Kegels

Choose the easiest position and perform a pelvic floor contraction as described on page 126. For endurance: work up to a 10-second hold, up to 10 times. Rest for 20 seconds if you are at risk of having too much tension.

For coordination/motor control: do quick flicks, up to 10 times in a row, with a clear contract/relax cycle of a second on, a second off.

Progress to endurance and motor control training in progressively difficult positions.

Tilt or lean forward with the Kegel to control the labia, vaginal/genital opening, and bladder.

Tilt or lean backward with the Kegel to control the coccyx and anal sphincter.

Sit or stand in neutral with the Kegel to train the perineum after a tear or episiotomy.

Introduction to the Pelvic Brace

This is the first step in building your pelvic brace—the rest can be found in chapter 8. You can practice this in any position, but we recommend sitting to start. Sit in anatomic neutral to be most aware of your perineum. Inhale down, allowing your ribs, belly, and pelvic floor to expand. Forcefully exhale, as though you are blowing out candles or breathing through a straw. During the exhale, Kegel. Once you are good at this, hold the Kegel while inhaling and exhaling again without losing control. This trains the pelvic floor to maintain control, even while you are breathing in and out. If you've been Kegeling by sucking in, you may lose control during the second inhalation. If you cannot do this, go back to regular Kegels, and be sure to perform them without inhaling or sucking in.

The Knack

Inhale down with the diaphragm. Then right before you exhale, Kegel, telling yourself that the bladder is lifting as well. Cough and hold the Kegel to reduce PFM pressure.

If you inhale up, sending your ribs toward the shoulders and neck, you will have to crash your ribs down into your belly to exhale, creating downward pressure on the bladder and pelvic floor. Inhaling down with your diaphragm ensures that the exhale will pull up, reducing bladder and PFM pressure.

Progress to standing, or in any position that tends to make you leak when you cough, laugh, and sneeze.

Reverse Kegels or Pelvic Floor Muscle Letdown

Practice relaxing the pelvic floor with a letdown. Try performing a brief (1 to 2 seconds) Kegel, then inhaling into the pelvic bowl until you feel a stretch in the pelvic floor. Enhance sensation by sitting on a washcloth or a large exercise ball. Try different positions. If you have constipation, practice in a seated or toilet position. If you have pain with sex, practice relaxing the pelvic floor in your favorite positions.

Happy Baby Pose

You may have done this one in yoga class. While lying on your back, bring one knee to your chest at a time, using your arms to brace the legs slightly apart. See if you can grab your ankles, the soles of your feet, or your big toes, and slowly hold the legs open with the knees bent. If you cannot, then hold your outer knees. Hold for 30 seconds and gently rock side to side. This pelvic floor opener can help you return to intercourse with your partner on top.

Prayer Squat

Stand with your legs wide apart and toes turned out. Make prayer hands in front of your chest with your palms together, elbows apart. Slowly squat down as low as you can, bringing your elbows to the insides of the knees, and dropping your hips toward the floor. This maximally lengthens your pelvic floor. Doing this requires full pelvic floor muscle letdown and a lot of mobility in your hips and pelvis. Completing this one without pain is a good sign that you're ready to return to penetrative intercourse with you positioned on top of your partner. If you are struggling, work on sitting on a low stool or yoga block. Work on getting the hips comfortable with being far apart. If you are still struggling, check out our next chapter, on the lumbopelvic system.

CHAPTER 7

The Lumbopelvic System

ANATOMY OF THE BUTTOCKS, HIPS, LUMBOSACRAL SPINE, AND PELVIS

The lumbopelvic system is the center of movement and stability in the human body, and it worked really hard to support both you and the baby. As your pregnancy progressed, these joints widened, and your center of gravity changed. But now that you are a single-person house again, that system needs to adapt. For some, the lumbopelvic system will resolve its changes on its own as you get back to more regular, unencumbered movement. For others, these shifts might persist for up to two years postpartum (according to our anecdotal observations). As the root of your foundational support system, the lumbopelvic system sets the stage for your sitting and standing posture. It transfers your body weight from your legs to your torso. It lets you bend, sit, stand, roll, lean, walk, climb, thrust, and twerk. What do all those things have in common? Movement. If this system is stable, then these movements will feel comfortable. If this system is unstable, they will be painful.

Bones, Joints, and Ligaments

Let's walk through the anatomy so you have a better understanding of the areas involved. The pelvis consists of three bones: the pubis in front, the ischium (sitz bones) on the bottom, and the ilium to the top and side. All three fuse at the acetabulum, or the socket of the hip joint. This is where the large leg bone (femur) inserts to form the hip joint. The sacrum, or the "butt bone," connects to the back of the pelvis. At the bottom of the sacrum is the coccyx, or tailbone, and the top connects the pelvis to the lumbar spine, or lower back.

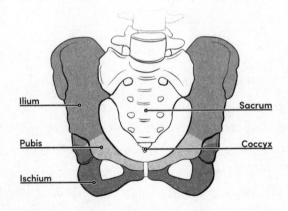

Ligaments and muscles hold your bones together at the joints. The left and right pubic bones come together with a cartilaginous "bumper" in between to form a joint called the symphysis pubis. The sacrum joins the pelvis to form the sacroiliac joints, one on each side. These bones can be prominent and feel like a small bump. The sacrum also connects to the low back to form the lumbosacral junction, buffered by the L5 vertebral disc. You might have heard this referred to as the L5/S1 (fifth lumbar and first sacral vertebrae). L5/S1 is where the sciatic nerve exits and travels down and outside of the sacrum into the buttock, extending down the back of the thigh.

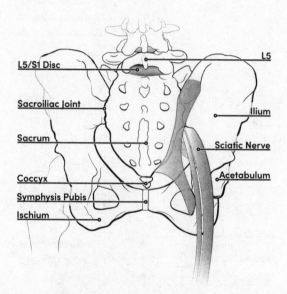

Muscles

The lumbopelvic system is intricately muscled, from the large and obvious gluteals to the buried iliopsoas. They coordinate to support your movement and stability.

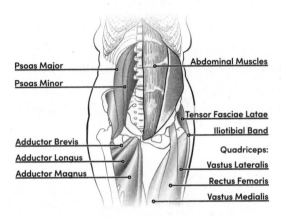

Psoas Major

Psoas Minor

Adductor Brevis

Adductor Longus

Adductor Magnus

Abdominal Muscles

Tensor Fasciae Latae

Iliotibial Band

Quadriceps:

Vastus Lateralis

Rectus Femoris

Vastus Medialis

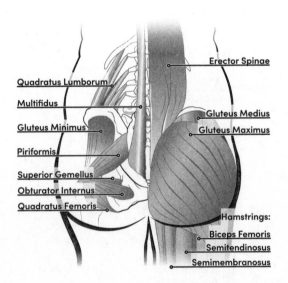

Quadratus Lumborum

Multifidus

Gluteus Minimus

Piriformis

Superior Gemellus

Obturator Internus

Quadratus Femoris

Erector Spinae

Gluteus Medius

Gluteus Maximus

Hamstrings:

Biceps Femoris

Semitendinosus

Semimembranosus

Muscles of the Lumbopelvic System

MUSCLES	WHERE ARE THEY?	WHAT DO THEY DO?
Pelvic floor (~20 total)	All over the bottom portion of the pelvis	Deep internal stability for organs and torso, sexual pleasure/arousal, control of closing and opening sphincters
Abdominals: rectus abdominis, internal obliques, external obliques, and transverse abdominis	Connecting ribs to pelvis and lumbar spine	Control your canister, protect your spine in rotation, hold your posture, support your organs
Deep back stabilizers: multifidus, quadratus lumborum, and transverse abdominis	Attaching spine to sacrum and iliac crest	Deep stabilizers to control spinal and pelvic motion, hold posture
Erector spinae	Connects to the spine along the length to the sacrum	Arches your back or bends it to one side
Iliopsoas, or the iliacus and the psoas (tip: the *p* is silent)	Bottom thoracic rib/spine and upper lumbar to inner groin (deep inside the belly)	Bends your hip, brings the body and leg closer together, turns the leg in
Groin/adductors	Inner femur, connecting the pubis to the femur	Pull the legs together, stabilize the hip in the socket
Gluteals: Gluteus maximus, gluteus medius, gluteus minimus	Your buttocks: top of the iliac crest to the sacrum and outer hip	Rotate and move the hip behind you or away from the body
Hip rotators: piriformis, obturator internus (also a PFM), obturator externus, gemellus superior and gemellus inferior, quadratus femoris	Wrapping around from the sacrum or ilium to the back of the femur	Stabilize the hip in the socket and rotate the hip out
Tensor fascia latae (TFL)	Connects the ilium to the outside of the femur, where it becomes the iliotibial band (IT band)	Assists in moving the leg away from the body

Muscles of the Lumbopelvic System

MUSCLES	WHERE ARE THEY?	WHAT DO THEY DO?
Quadriceps and rectus femoris	Connect pelvis to front of the femur and cross the knee	Straighten the knee and lift the leg forward
Hamstrings	Connect the ischium or sitz bones to the posterior thigh all the way to the lower leg below the knee	Bend the knee and pull the leg behind you

Common musculoskeletal conditions of the postpartum pelvis are symphysis pubis dysfunction (SPD), sacroiliac (SI) joint pain, lumbar spine pain, sciatica, or hip pain. We are going to call this entire phenomenon pelvic girdle pain (PGP). About a quarter of postpartum people experience PGP in the first six weeks. It often resolves by week 12, but it can persist for up to two years, and evidence suggests that those who had a cesarean birth will have more pain than those who had a vaginal/genital delivery. Your risk is increased if you had pain prior to pregnancy, have a BMI higher than 25, had pelvic girdle pain in pregnancy, experienced depression in pregnancy, or worked a physically demanding job while pregnant. Hypermobility or hypermobile-type Ehlers Danlos syndrome can also increase your risk of PGP lasting beyond twelve weeks.

PELVIC GIRDLE PAIN

Pelvic girdle pain can negatively impact your mental and physical well-being. The lumbopelvic region is central to your stability and movement, so if it hurts, it will make the basic acts of living hard to do. This leaves people angry, frustrated, irritable, and sometimes physically unable to care for themselves or their families.

Resolving Pelvic Girdle Pain

Pelvic girdle pain can feel like muscle tightness, so your instinct might be to try to stretch. But the ligaments in your pelvis stretched during pregnancy, so more stretching isn't the answer. The feeling of tightness is often caused by muscles like the hamstring or psoas being recruited to do work without help from your deep stabilizing core system. Gaining strength and stability in the lumbopelvic system is the key to resolving most pelvic girdle pain.

SACROILIITIS,
OR SI JOINT DYSFUNCTION

The SI joint gets angry when it moves too much or is hypermobile. Both SI joints should work together to shift your weight left and right or up and down through the pelvis. If one side moves too much, it can cause inflammation that leads to pain and poor muscle activation, usually called sacroiliitis. SI joint pain is typically worse when standing on one leg, going up stairs, or rolling over in bed. The issue could be internal to the sacrum, meaning it has tilted or torqued. Vaginal/genital tearing on one side can make this more likely, as it causes the pelvic floor to pull unevenly on the sacrum. You might benefit from knowing if you tore centrally or left and right; ask your provider if you're unsure. Focus on tightening the weaker side of the pelvic floor or getting the core, glutes, and adductors to help support the pelvis until your tear heals.

Issues with the SI joint could also be caused by the ilium shifting to a new position—either up, down, out, or in from pelvic neutral. Working on neutral pelvic posture when sitting and standing or carrying things—including a baby—on both sides of the body more or less equally will stop the problem from getting worse. Try wearing a sacroiliac joint stabilizing belt if all movements are painful.

You may get relief with joint manipulation from an osteopath, PT, or chiropractor, but those adjustments won't provide lasting relief if the real issue is muscle weakness or lopsided posture. Avoid exercises that "over-stretch" the SI joint, such as pigeon pose in yoga, low lunges, lunges, deep squats, hamstring stretches, or heavy single-leg work, or any time one leg is far in front of your body and the other is far behind you. You can return to those things in small increments once you know your pelvic floor has healed, and you can do the below exercises regularly without pain.

Exercises for SI Relief

Gluteal Activation

The glutes act together to pull on the sacrum and the ilium in relation to the hip joint. Check for gluteal activation by squeezing one buttock at a time while lying down. You might use your hand to feel the contraction. It should be robust and equal on both sides. Often the side with dysfunction and pain will be weaker with less bulk and fullness when you squeeze it. The treatment is to keep checking in and getting the glutes turned on. Pay attention to the rest of the system. Are you tightening your back instead of your butt? Do you have to tilt your pelvis, or can you keep your joints and bones still? You should be keeping them still. You can squeeze your glutes in any position, including standing. Focus on getting the weaker side to activate by putting weight on it. Many people avoid putting weight into sore joints, which can lead to increased weakness by lack of use. Load the joint and squeeze it so you can learn to stabilize it comfortably. Isometrics tend to make people do weird things with their breath. Make sure you are exhaling with the exertion, not locking your throat, inhaling, or clenching your abs.

Pelvic Reset

With the help of a willing partner, lie on your back, bend your knees, and place your feet and knees together. Have your partner wrap their arms around your knees (or wrap your thighs above the knee with a yoga strap/belt). Push out into your partner's arms as if to separate your knees. Make sure your partner knows that they should *not* let you win. Push up to 10 seconds, 1 to 3 repetitions only. Then separate your knees, keeping them bent and your feet together. Your partner should put their forearm—or you can use a ball or yoga block—between your thighs near the knee but not on the knee joint. Squeeze your thighs together as hard as you can up to 10 seconds and 3 repetitions. You may hear or feel your pubic bone pop; don't worry. If you feel too much pressure at your pubic bone, use the heel of your hand on top for stabilization to generate the necessary muscle force. The adductors are activating to stabilize the SI joints and symphysis pubis.

Sacral Reset

Lie on your back with your knees bent and place a soft four-inch ball (not a lacrosse ball or tennis ball) at the center of your sacrum. Put your body weight on it. You might feel immediate pain if your sacrum is not in neutral. Try to relax into the ball, breathe into your belly and pelvic floor, and let your muscle tension go for 1 to 5 minutes as tolerated. Do not persist if you are having a lot of pain.

Ball and Band

The pelvic reset turns into a gentle strengthening exercise with the help of a resistance band or yoga belt and a ball or rolled-up large towel. Place the band around your thighs just above your knees. Gently press your thighs apart into the band. Do not go as far as you possibly can, only as far as you can while keeping your feet flat and ankles together. Do not push into hip or pelvic pain, either. Repeat 10 to 30 times. Follow up

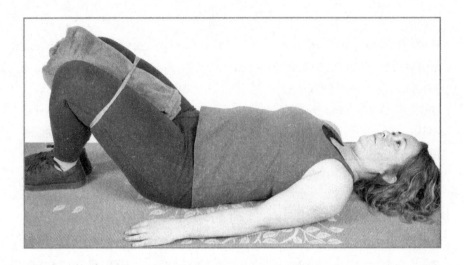

with an inner thigh squeeze against a 6-inch ball or rolled-up towel, 10 to 30 reps. The pelvis should not tilt with these exercises. You can practice a gentle exhale with any exerting force to keep from bearing down.

Controlled Walking

Brisk walking for 20 to 30 minutes can reduce SI joint pain. Monitor your stride, taking small but controlled steps rather than letting your step length exceed your pelvic stability, which can create downward pressure on the SI joint, increasing laxity and inflammation. Roll smoothly from an initial heel contact to your toes with every step. Your footfalls should be quiet, not heavy. If this is painful, try it with a sacroiliac stabilizing belt.

SPD: SYMPHYSIS PUBIS DYSFUNCTION

SPD is pain where the pubic bones meet. This often starts during pregnancy or begins after a vaginal/genital delivery. The pain begins in the pubis and radiates to the front of the pelvis or down into the groin. You may feel or hear concerning popping sounds from the pubis. Generally, we associate this with too much separation or poor alignment of the two pubic bones to that cartilaginous bumper in the center. The pain typically worsens when doing things that separate the legs, like getting out of the car, getting out of bed, or stepping over a baby gate. Modify your movements to reduce leg separation, including keeping your legs together when getting in and out of bed or a car, refraining from sexual experiences that encourage the legs to be wide apart, and avoiding wide-legged yoga poses or stretches. When you sit for prolonged periods, including for feeding a baby, make sure you are in a chair that allows the legs to be together without needing to sit cross-legged. Do not sit on the floor, as every way you want to get up could be straining, even if the sitting is comfortable.

Exercises for SPD Relief

Groin Squeezes

Sitting in a chair or lying on your back with knees bent, squeeze a ball or rolled towel with a strong but comfortable effort. Hold 5 to 10 seconds. Repeat 10 times. Do as needed when acute pain occurs.

Groin Squeezes as a Retraining

Lie on your side with your knees bent to about 60 degrees and feet together, hips stacked neutrally with your pointy pelvic bone (anterior superior iliac spine, or ASIS) pointed forward, not up at the ceiling. Place a foam roller, stack of pillows, or bolster between your feet and knees. Gently squeeze your top groin muscle. This should pull the top knee into the bottom knee. If you cannot contract your groin or inner thigh, you will notice the psoas and tensor fasciae latae (TFL) pop out near your ASIS, or that your pelvis tilts. Try sticking your butt out a little behind you or using a larger stack between the knees to get the groin working. Hold 5 to 10 seconds and repeat up to 10 times on each side.

Pelvic Tilts

Lying on your back, perform a pelvic brace and tilt your pubic bone up toward your ribs. Remember that is a pull to midline, exhale, and lift of the pelvic floor muscle with the lower abdominals. This can be done seated on a large (65 centimeter) exercise ball or in hands and knees position. You want to create pressure from the bottom up. Do up to 20 in a comfortable range of motion.

Progression 1: Add a glute squeeze at the top of the tilt. This should help tuck the buttocks under slightly, increasing the tilt.

Progression 2: While lying on your back, push down through your feet and press up into a bridge. Again, make sure your core is on first, glutes second, and hamstrings third. Don't arch your back and lift from the ribs.

Pelvic Floor Exercises

With any activity that hurts your symphysis pubis, try using a pelvic brace before you move: Exhale, activate your lower abs and pelvic floor, hold that tension, then move.

BACK PAIN

Postpartum back pain is usually linked to too much tension in the multifidus, erector spinae, psoas, and quadratus lumborum. It can also involve compression of the discs in the lumbar spine. The back muscles are likely showing up most for you during daily movements, making them tight, tense, and overworked.

If you have back pain and numbness, tingling, or weakness in your legs, your legs are giving way, you have pain that does not go away no matter what position you are in, your pain keeps you up at night, and/or you lose bowel and bladder control, seek medical attention. Those are all red flags that you could have a severe spinal injury and should get medical help immediately.

Otherwise, the best thing you can do for back pain caused by a muscle imbalance is walk. Walking 20 to 30 minutes at a comfortable pace without pushing or carrying anything or anyone can help you get enough muscle activation, load bearing, rotation, breathing, and blood flow to calm down any muscle spasms that are contributing to your pain. Bed rest and movement avoidance are not recommended, as your pain will feel worse when you try to move or change position and your muscles will get weaker and tighter. If you must stay in one position for a long time, your back will be happiest with neutral spine and pelvic posture. Get your feet on the floor. If you are short, bring the floor to your feet with a stool. Use a back rest so you aren't becoming rigid during the day. Use a small rolled towel behind your lower back for more support, and apply heat or ice to take the edge off your pain.

Recliners are bad news for disc pain. A recliner lets you get into posterior pelvic tilt with a flexed spine, which allows herniated disc material to increase pressure back toward your spinal column and nerves. Because flexion reduces pressure on your discs, you don't feel it happening when you're in the recliner. As you get up and load your spine again, it hits you like, WHAM! Big pain. Can't stand up straight. Can't walk. Potentially increased pain, numbness, and tingling down the leg. Find seats that are straighter in the back. When your back gets tired of being straight, walk or lie down.

Decompression for Positional Relief

To resolve back pain, first identify which positions offer you relief and don't make your back feel worse afterward. Spend 10 to 20 minutes here at least two times a day (but do not sleep in these positions). We have two favorites.

Prone over Pillows

Lie facedown, using pillows under your belly to reduce chest/breast pressure if you're lactating. Stack your hands beneath your forehead and put pillows underneath the lower part of your legs and tops of your feet so your hamstrings aren't pulling at your pelvis. Add rolled towels under your shoulders if you need more chest support. Practice breathing here. Expand your posterior ribs to let them move with more ease. Practice gluteal squeezes here to stabilize your pelvis.

Advanced: Positional wedges underneath the anterior superior iliac spine or the pelvis can assist with more bony support and pelvic neutral. Being in pelvic neutral can "reset" your system, which reduces spasms and improves your ability to find this position more often. Look up "wedge positioners" or flip some hard-bottomed clogs or sneakers over and put them in toe side first. They work just as well.

Decompression in 90/90

This position places your hips and knees at 90 degrees. Its purpose is to reduce pressure on the vertebrae and discs through positional traction to offer relief from compression. If you're in a lot of spasm, this might be uncomfortable at first, but should feel better in 3 to 5 minutes. Lie on your back on your bed or the floor and place your lower legs on an object like a large exercise ball, an upside-down laundry basket, or a chair that lets you get close to a 90-degree bend in your hips and knees. The height should be comfortable, and your lower legs should be parallel to the bed or floor. Breathe here, allowing your arms to go anywhere they feel comfortable. Focus on breathing into any areas that feel tight or in spasm. Let the bones in your body get heavier, relaxing down into the surface more with time.

Focus on the basics of pain management. Rest intermittently during your day to reduce the muscles in spasm or increasing tension. Use an active range of motion and take movement opportunities that don't worsen your pain (although you might still hurt). Walk every day as if it is your highest priority. We know you have many demands on your time, so enlist your community of care to get this to happen. Do stabilizing exercises as listed above for the other pelvic health conditions. Try the exercises from chapter 8, "The Core," once you feel more stable.

If you still don't feel stable, try a brace or lumbosacral stabilizing orthoses, which are almost all corset style. If you can get a diagnosis that is covered by insurance from a doctor and a referral to physical therapy, the PT can often order the brace, in which case your insurance will pay for it, and you may be able to try on different models to see what gives you relief. If you cannot go through that process, order one online. You'll be asked to submit a measurement around your hips. The goal of the brace is to allow you to move more during your day and get your daily tasks done. Wear the brace when you are performing movement tasks that cause back pain, not when you're sitting, sleeping, or resting.

SCIATICA

Sciatica is pain in the sciatic nerve caused by compression, inflammation, or irritation. The sciatic nerve has origins from the spinal cord at levels L4 to S3 and merges to form the largest peripheral nerve in the human body. You have one on either side. The nerve exits next to the sacrum into the buttock, typically near the largest hip rotator muscle, the piriformis. It then travels down the back of the leg along with the hamstrings. Once it nears the knee, it divides and is renamed. The sciatic nerve tells your hamstrings and part of your groin muscles what to do, and interprets sensation in your lower leg, particularly the top of the foot into the first and second toes.

Symptoms of sciatica are pain in the buttock that radiates down the leg, with or without numbness and tingling in the same areas. If compressed, it will cause weakness of the hamstrings and groin. If it's just irritated, you will have pain. A severe symptom of sciatica could be foot drop, which is the inability to control lifting your foot up. Definitely go see a doctor if you have this.

A small percentage of postpartum sciatica can be caused by positioning during your cesarean birth, the amount of time you spent pushing while on your back, an infection of the uterus, or a fracture in your sacrum. Sciatica is more common in folks with endometriosis and tends to be right-sided and congruent with your menstrual cycle or inflammation. It can also be caused by a disc bulge between L3 and S1 or the piriformis muscle entrapping the nerve.

Postpartum sciatica is treated similarly to back pain: don't overload your body, take walks, and work on pelvic stability. You can add some piriformis and hamstring stretching and getting your uterus off your spine to the mix.

Piriformis Stretching

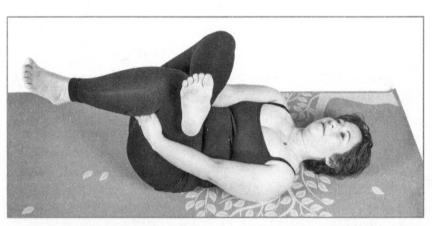

Lie on your back and bend both knees. Cross one ankle over the other knee. Grasp the leg that is bent but not crossed and pull it toward your body (never push on the crossed knee). Hold to your comfort. When stretching muscles near nerves, avoid irritating the nerve, as it can cause more symptoms, so ease up if it feels painful. Hold 30 seconds and repeat 3 times. Test both sides to see if there is a difference in comfort or range of motion.

Adaptation: Sit and cross one ankle over the knee, gently leaning forward. Keep your back straight and hinge from the hips instead of rounding the back forward.

Adaptation 2: Pull the crossed knee toward the opposite shoulder.

Pet Peeve Alert: Ruth has a lot of patients with chronic sciatica who have been told to push a small hard ball, like a tennis, lacrosse, or massage ball, into their buttocks to relieve the pain. The problem with this, of course, is pushing a hard ball into a nerve is painful. It can *cause* irritation. Then when it hurts more, people push the ball into their nerves more, creating a negative feedback loop. The premise of this treatment is the belief that if you dig into something painful, it will get better. Most people are aiming for their piriformis muscle here but aren't skilled enough or taught enough to know the difference between nerve pain and what a muscle in spasm feels like. If the muscle is so tight it entraps the nerve, move the muscle more. Stretch your piriformis and go for a walk. Beating it into submission will only cause more trauma.

Hamstring Stretching

Sit on the edge of a hard surface. Straighten one knee so that the heel is on the ground, the knee is straight, and the spine is stacked over the pelvis. The other knee is bent to 90 degrees, with the foot flat on the ground. You should be balanced equally on your sitz bones. Maintain a straight spine, and hinge at the hips to feel a stretch down the back of the leg. Hold this stretch without bouncing for 30 to 60 seconds and repeat 3 times on either side. If your sciatic nerve is sensitive, "flossing" it by pumping your ankle at the end of the stretch can reduce pain and sensitivity (even if it zings a little during the action).

Getting Your Uterus off Your Spine

Get on your hands and knees. Breathe and let your belly drop. Don't tuck your butt under. Stay here for up to eight breaths. That's it! If you'd like, add some cat/cows and rock-backs to improve spinal mobility.

Generally, any nerve pain whose origin is spinal will have a natural timeline for healing. The main goal is not irritating the condition further. Regular movement, good posture, heat/ice, medications that are approved by your doctor, and time are the best treatments. If you find certain activities make the pain travel down the leg, stop those. If the pain is traveling a shorter distance down your leg, that's a good sign that there is less pressure on your nerve.

HIP PAIN

Hip pain not described by anything else in this chapter is typically from pregnancy-related muscle imbalances. It tends to get worse with side-lying, extended periods of sitting, or extended periods of walking. It's a smaller part of the larger "pelvic girdle pain" complex and can be caused by the hormone changes in pregnancy that cause lower bone density or tears in the ligaments that hold the hip in place. Not being able to tolerate any weight on your leg is a red flag that should send you to medical diagnostics to see what's going on.

Lateral Pelvic Shift

Standing in neutral posture, legs wider than hip distance apart, shift your pelvis to one side until you feel a stretch. Depending on where your hips are tight, you might feel a stretch on the outside of the hip or the inner groin, or both. Hold 30 seconds and do 3 reps. Repeat on both sides.

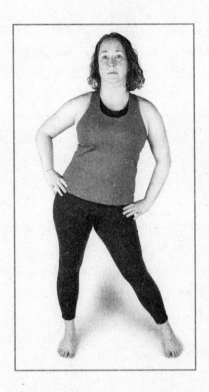

Quadratus Lumborum Stretch

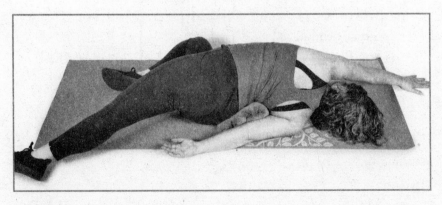

Lie on your side with one to two pillows between your ribs and your pelvis. Straighten your top leg and move it behind you. Stretch the top arm away from the top leg, rolling the upper body forward and the lower body backward. This should stretch the space between the ribs and the pelvis. Hold up to 1 minute. Repeat on the tighter side.

Standing Hip Hikes and Drops

Standing on the ground, hold your pelvis with your hands. Hike one side of the pelvis up, pushing the opposite leg into the ground. This will shorten the space between the ribs and pelvis on the hiked-up side. Repeat 10 times each side.

Advanced: This uses the same concept, but drop the leg off a step as far as you can and hike it as high as you can.

Advanced 2: Complete a neutral pelvis step-up from the side. The higher the step, the harder it is to hold neutral. Repeat 10 times to start. Increase sets as tolerated.

A Few Old Favorites

Glute sets to balance and stabilize your hips.

Kegels, because they are part of your deep core and will help you stay in postural neutral.

Groin squeezes to activate your deep core and stabilize your pelvis.

IMPORTANT HIP MECHANICS

Glutes

Your glutes are major players in pelvic stability. They help keep your back muscles from working too much and becoming sore and tight, they keep your postpartum pelvis from tipping too far anterior (arched low back), and they are the primary stabilizers for the SI joints. Glute strength will keep you moving comfortably as your core and pelvic floor heal in the postpartum period by reducing pelvic girdle pain, retraining posterior pelvic floor mechanics, and helping you maintain fecal continence (as in not pooping your pants!).

It's tempting to jump right back into squats, lunges, fire hydrants, bird dogs, or donkey kicks. These exercises are great if you're already stable and don't have other back, ankle, or core deficits. But if you're not stable, these exercises can be challenging or can cause joint pain. Postpartum people and folks who are hypermobile can tend to overuse back extensors. This can happen in any exercise that pushes the leg behind the body. Make sure that you know the goal of the exercises you are trying and that you are activating the glutes when you should be.

Beware of overclenching the gluteals, too. Strike a balance between tension and relaxation, just as with your pelvic floor. An overclenched butt is tucked under all the time, including when sitting and standing, with hips pressed forward and weight into the balls of the feet. This is sometimes referred to as "mom butt" (cringe!).

The tucked butt originates in pregnancy. As your pregnant belly gets heavier, it becomes difficult to hinge at the hips, since you might fall over. To compensate, you lead with your buttocks to get out of a chair instead of leaning forward with your torso. You start to push your hips into counters to stabilize instead of using your core. Your shirt is wet after doing dishes. This movement pattern requires retraining. It just takes practice—and a willingness to overcome any nagging voices telling us not to stick our butts out.

One of the tasks of the gluteal muscles is to lengthen to allow you to hinge again from your hips. This movement pattern allows you to get up from a seated position and to lift things from the floor in a way that protects your back and utilizes the deep core system.

Hip Hinge

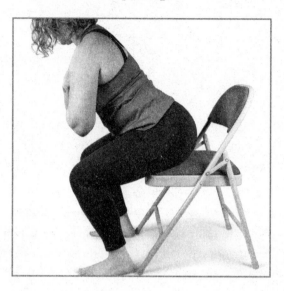

Sit on the edge of a chair with your feet flat on the ground. Cross your arms over your chest and lean forward with a straight back, keeping your knees in line with your toes and your pelvis neutral. Try to feel the moment when your weight transfers from your buttocks to your feet. In a good hip hinge, this is exactly what happens. This is the moment that your gluteals are responsible for handling your body weight and pushing it up to stand. Practice holding this deep hinge for 10 seconds while breathing fully.

Progression 1: Stand with legs slightly wider than hip distance apart and knees gently bent. Hinge at the hips, leaning forward with a neutral spine. Your glutes should lengthen. In other words, your bottom should be sticking out. This is a great place to practice *inhale down and blow up!* Inhale into the hinge and blow up to stand.

Progression 2: Add weights to your hip hinge to progressively load your glutes and hamstrings to be longer and stronger. You should be able to do 10 reps without pain.

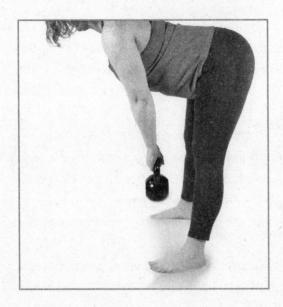

If the back of your thighs feels tight, spend time increasing inner thigh mobility.

Kickstand Rock-Back

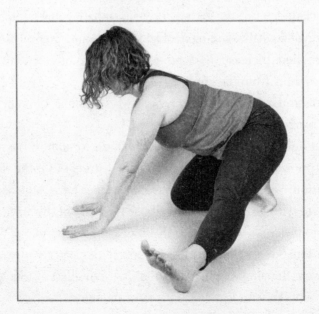

Get on your hands and knees. Kick one leg out to the side with a straight knee. Balance the weight of your leg on the heel. Gently stick your butt out and shift your body weight toward your heels. You will feel inner thigh tension. Try this in repeats of 10 instead of long holds. Check both sides.

Lateral Step-Ups

Stand perpendicular to a stool, step, or stair. Place one foot on the step. Lean forward in a hip hinge (back straight; ankle, knee, and hip bent). Shift weight to the stepped-up leg and generate pressure in that leg by pushing hard into the foot. This should result in a step-up. Hover at the top. Restart.

For an extra challenge, after you hover, return the foot to the ground by bending your ankle, knee, and hip as slowly and carefully as you can.

Squats

Stand with feet hip distance apart, toes slightly turned out. Bend ankles, knees, and hips with a straight back to squat down. Squat as low as you can without causing your arches to drop, your knees to turn in, or your butt to tuck under. Breathe for integration by inhaling down into the squat and blowing up when standing. Hold 5 to 10 seconds. Repeat 10 times.

Progression: Increase the depth of the squat to be able to touch and/or lift something from the ground.

Progression 2: Perform with a weight—for example, dumbbells, a kettlebell, a plate weight.

Regression: Hold on to a sink or door handle to support the squat and your posture while you rebuild leg and spinal strength for the squat.

Variation: Squat with your legs close together for a "suitcase" squat. Squat down with a straight back, and use the bend of the ankles, knees, and hips to pick up a weight from the floor with one hand.

Variation: Squat with your legs far apart, toes slightly turned out for a sumo squat. If using weights, hold them to your chest or touch them to the floor between your legs at the depth of the squat.

Hip Flexors

We have bundles of hip flexor muscles on either side of the body, which pull the body and femur toward each other. The psoas is the largest and often the most problematic hip flexor, because it tends to shorten during pregnancy and can end up in spasm. Hip flexor spasms are felt as pain in the front of the belly, pelvis, groin, or anterior thigh. They can also present as back pain or a stomachache. They tend to get worse with prolonged sitting or prolonged walking. Knowing if you have issues with these muscles can be tricky; as Ruth usually tells her patients, "You can't get there from here" to massage them easily.

A shortened psoas can pull the femur forward in its socket, followed by the obturator internus and piriformis muscles, which lock it in place. Activating the glutes and the groin and adductor muscles of the inner thigh will help shut this pattern down, as will allowing your butt to stick out, rather than tuck under, when standing.

Exercises to Balance the Hip Rotators

Bridges

Lie on your back with your knees bent. Activate your glutes and exhale to brace the pelvis. Push into your heels to activate your hamstrings. Using these muscles will allow you to perform this exercise with a stable pelvis without recruiting your psoas and back muscles. Roll your pelvis up from the bottom by continuing to push into your feet. Don't arch your back or lift your ribs. Hold 5 to 10 seconds as you breathe slowly. Stop if you experience spasm in the legs or pelvic girdle pain. Gradually build up your endurance until you can hold the bridge position for 60 seconds.

Progression: Bridging with a march. In the bridge, hold your trunk neutral while decreasing leg support. You will need to hold a gentle pelvic brace and cue yourself to keep breathing without locking the throat. Start by lifting one heel and replacing it, then the other. The goal is to remain in pelvic neutral without the hips dropping when the foot lifts. Progress to lift the whole foot up without tilting the pelvis or spine.

Progression: Bridging with a straight leg raise. In a bridge, keep your thighs parallel. Slowly lift one foot off the ground and straighten the leg at the knee, keeping your thighs parallel and your pelvis and spine neutral. Breathe without bearing down. This is very hard to do! Hold 5 seconds, and repeat 5 times. Repeat the whole sequence straightening the other leg. This will be easier on you if you alternate sides. Because exercise math can be tricky, count right leg *one*, left leg *two* . . . up to 10, to complete 5 on each side.

Once you are good at this, upgrade to pushing from the ground with one leg straight and one leg bent (runners, this is for you!).

Modified Bird Dogs

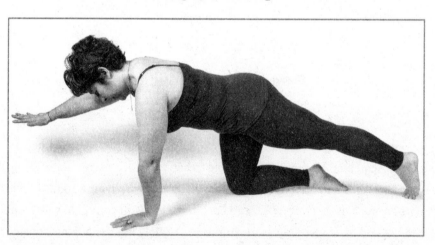

In a tabletop position on your hands and knees, perform a pelvic brace. Slowly slide one leg backward, keeping the toes on the ground, like a plank, extending the opposite arm parallel to the ground at shoulder height. Hold and feel for your glutes and core to be on and your back straight without twisting or curling. Return to hands and knees. Repeat 5 times on each side.

Variation: When this becomes easy and not wobbly, after you slide your leg backward, lift it off the ground in line with the torso. Remember not to arch your spine. You should feel your glutes and core working to stop you from rotating.

Monster Walks

Tie a resistance band around your feet (this better targets your glutes than a band around the thighs would) at shoulder width apart. Squat slightly, with ankles, knees, and hips bent. Stay in the mini-squat and step to the side, keeping your toes forward. Walk 10 feet to one side and then 10 feet to the other. Make sure you don't accidentally stand up straighter as you walk. Stay in the mini-squat.

Straight Leg Series

This works the hip and knee against gravity in all directions. The goal is to learn to brace your pelvis, spine, and abs with coordination during leg movements. Watch your core pressure and breathing here. Tell yourself to "pull your bladder up" if your belly is bulging or your pelvic floor feels heavy. Do only as many reps as you can with good total form: posture, diaphragm, abs, pelvic floor, and leg stability. If you have one side that is clearly not as strong or doing as well as the other, do more sets on that side to promote balance.

1. **Flexion:** Lying on your back with both knees bent, straighten one leg and hold it with the thighs parallel to each other. Hold 5 seconds and slowly lower the leg back down. Bend the knee and repeat 10 times. The more slowly you lower the leg, the more control you need from your core. Repeat the sequence on the other side.

2. **Abduction:** Lying on your side in pelvic neutral, straighten the top knee and lift it up about 6 inches only. Repeat 10 times on one side. Then repeat the sequence on the other side.

3. **Adduction:** Lying on your side in pelvic neutral, bend the top leg and use it as a tripod, bending at hip and knee and placing the foot in front of the bottom straight leg. Lift the bottom straight leg up 3 inches, then lower. Do 10 reps. Then repeat the sequence on the other side.

4. **Extension:** Lie on your stomach (pad underneath with pillows if you have a large arch in your lower back or need to support your chest). Perform a pelvic brace connecting the pubic bone to ribs and activating core support. Do a one-sided glute set, slowly lifting your straight leg up behind you without arching your back. Do 10 reps. Then repeat the sequence on the other side. If you cannot do this without arching your back, go back to modified bird dogs and regular glute sets for a while.

Band Corrections for Hip

1. **Forward walk/lunge:** This exercise is to help people with a dominant anterior hip, TFL, or psoas. Take a resistance band, loop it, and anchor it in a doorway or to a stable gym surface. Step into the loop with the weaker or more painful leg, bringing the edge of the band to the front of your hip. Face away from the surface or doorway. Take small steps forward, allowing the band to pull you back. Once you feel tension on the band, anchor the banded leg, foot facing straight ahead, pelvis and spine neutral. Step the un-banded leg forward into a mini-lunge: front leg ahead, back leg straight. Then step back. Stay strong in your stance. Only step as far as you can with control. As the front step lengthens, the back heel rises. This should help you feel the glutes turn on and pull the femur back.

2. **Side walk/squat:** This exercise is to help people with a one-sided pelvic tilt, chronic baby hip, or chronic buttock/hip pain. Take a strong resistance band, loop it, and anchor in a doorway or stable gym surface. Step into the loop with one leg, bringing the edge of the band to the groin. Step away from the door so the loop pulls on your groin more. Take side steps away from the door, allowing the band to pull on the groin as much as tolerated. Once you've reached the end of your tether, shift your pelvis to the side, doing a lateral pelvic tilt. You can also perform a mini-squat here. Check both sides and perform more sets on the tighter side.

IN THIS CHAPTER:

ANATOMY

CORE TRAINING CONSIDERATIONS

DOES A WEAK CORE REALLY CAUSE BACK PAIN?

OVERTENSING THE ABS

DIGESTION-RELATED ABDOMINAL CONSIDERATIONS

LINKING THORACIC SPINE AND RIBS TO CORE FUNCTION

HOW TO FIRE UP YOUR BEST CORE

BRACING SUPPORTS
LUMBOSACRAL STABILIZING ORTHOSIS (LSO)
BINDERS AND SHAPERS

CORE EXERCISES
CHIN-TUCK HEAD LIFT
PELVIC BRACE
ISOMETRIC OBLIQUES
DEAD BUG PROGRESSIONS
FRONT PLANKS
SIDE PLANKS
BIRD DOG PROGRESSIONS

CHAPTER 8

The Core

What can you expect from your postpartum abdominals? Well, they will be weaker anywhere from six to twelve weeks postpartum and return to baseline by twelve months. The muscles will have a thinner cross section and become more easily fatigued for four to six months. About two-thirds of you will have a separation in the front wall of the abdominals, called a diastasis recti (see chapter 2 for a refresher). For half of you with a DR, it's likely to reduce within twelve months. Reduce can mean the distance is not as far or the depth of the tissue separation is less. While DR has made a lot of waves in social media and online forums, the medical industry is still deciding if this is just a cosmetic deficit or something that requires intervention. People in the pelvic health industry are continuing to push for research to ascertain if your DR is linked to pelvic floor dysfunction, back pain, and other health conditions.

For folks with a cesarean birth, your abdominal muscles have been separated and you will have uterine scarring that limits how comfortable you are during exercise and movements that use abdominal activation for stabilization. There is no timeline for this. The eight-week postpartum checkup will determine if your scar is closed and your risk of infection is lower. It will not determine the status of your scar tissue beyond its initial closure. It will not determine how much pressure, weight, load, or repetition your scar can take. Doing too much too soon will strain your scar, and you will have to recover before you can load the tissues again comfortably and without symptoms. This will necessarily slow you down; otherwise it can lead to injury.

Core recovery following cesarean birth requires intentionality and continuing the scar massage work (chapter 2) for a while. How long is a while? Until you aren't getting those signals from your stomach, scar, bladder, pelvic floor, or back that loading, weight, and repetition are painful and heavy after doing work. For those of you who carried twins, the amount of stretching your abdominals went through will take more time to recover. It is essential to muscle recovery and function that you load your abdominals, but with all these considerations, how you do that will likely look different from what you were doing before pregnancy.

There is not yet enough research and consensus on how to handle every core deficit, no matter your delivery method or whether you have DR. When the research says "return to baseline," we are not even sure what those metrics are and how they relate to you in your life. Many times, it's just "not bleeding" or no "measurable deficit." There is a lot of variability to what anyone considers their baseline. Stay tuned in with your body as it is now, and with any future pregnancy or any change in your health status. Be honest and true to your current abilities to reduce the risk of further injury. More is not better. Harder is not better. *Smarter* is better.

ANATOMY

What is the anatomy of the core, and why aren't we just saying abdominals or abs? The core is a functional movement system that controls pressure in the torso and protects it. This includes the four layers of abdominal muscle: the rectus abdominis (RA), the external obliques (EO), the internal obliques (IO), and the transverse abdominis (TA). It includes muscles that support your lower back, specifically a group called the multifidus/multifidi. It also includes your pelvic floor and diaphragm. Skeletally, it includes your pelvis; your thoracic, lumbar, and sacral spine; and your ribs.

A postpartum core is often too loose in the front and too tight in the back, and can struggle to create enough tension to support you and your organs from below. A postpartum core will not do as good a job lifting each vertebra away from the others, causing a mild compression in the discs. This can make you feel like you want to slouch all the time. You may notice all of this as a general sag on your torso, which is likely to get worse as your activity increases or as the day goes on. Evening may bring heaviness, weakness, and soreness until you recover to a new level of strength and conditioning.

CORE TRAINING CONSIDERATIONS

Training your core needs to be slow because it requires your full attention not to fall into bad movement patterns. There is no perfect core exercise; there is simply the one that you can start with to get an isometric contraction that turns on your whole system. This could happen in any position, but partial resting positions are easiest, like lying down with supports (decompression) or sitting and resting your back on a seat. It is not reasonable or recommended to pull your belly in all the time; that is not a core contraction, that is a drawing-in maneuver. You can tell a drawing-in maneuver because the ribs are prominent, but the lower belly is not pulled in or contracted very well. Although a drawing-in maneuver is a viable stabilization strategy for a weak body, it's also an incomplete strategy that will fail under high loads and complex movements. For the postpartum person, it can increase downward pressure on the pelvic floor and pelvic organs, leading to leakage and prolapse (this would be much worse for anyone with a perineal or levator laceration from vaginal/genital delivery, or episiotomy). It can increase intra-abdominal pressure to the discs in the spine, putting you at higher risk for herniation. If your diaphragm and abs remain weak, it can lead to an abdominal wall or hiatal hernia. It can make it so that you can contract your core only if you are holding your breath, meaning that once the breath is used for something else, you are unstable in your body. It's not sustainable for regular daily movements.

A basic core contraction happens in spinal neutral, with a gentle exhale breath, a gentle wrapping around the torso between ribs and pelvis, and a gentle uplift as if sliding your belly button closer to the rib cage. Ensure you aren't bearing down into your healing pelvic organs. Use your fingers to see if you can feel the muscles one inch inside the ASIS (the front pokey pelvic bones) on the abdomen become a little bit taut. You should not be able to sink all the way to your guts with your fingers. Filming yourself during a core contraction can also provide useful feedback. Make sure the contraction is not all upper abdominals pulling the ribs down, with the lower belly protruding (external oblique dominant pattern), central abdominal bulge (rectus abdominis dominant pattern), or tight upper belly and flabby lower belly (diaphragm inhale up without deep core activation pattern). Try thinking about contracting from the bottom up, pubic bone to rib cage, to retrain the transverse abdominis and internal obliques to recruit again.

Focus on activation first, quickly contracting and then fully releasing the core. Repeat until you're fatigued or unable to get the right sequence of contraction and release. Once that is easy, practice holding a little bit of tension in the abdominal wall while inhaling and exhaling. This will ensure you are not stuck in a breath-holding pattern.

DOES A WEAK CORE
REALLY CAUSE BACK PAIN?

Imagine you just had a cesarean birth and you're going to try to lift a ten-pound object. Ouch! Your stomach and incision really hurt. To compensate, you lean back, pushing your stomach out. (In fact you might do that anyway; it's a habit held over from pregnancy.) This loads the spine more than any other part of your core and trains your spinal muscles to tense up more than your abs. They will quickly get tight and painful from overuse and overtension. Leaning back will feel easier than standing up straight, and because being postpartum is exhausting, you are going to do that when you're not thinking about it.

The other thing that is missing here is spinal disc support. Good core contractions lift the vertebrae away from one another and give your discs more room to move. The transverse abdominus (TA), sometimes confusingly called the lower abs (lower in depth in the body, not in distance to the pelvis), is most responsible for this support system. The TA is elusive, because it's most closely linked with the PFM (pelvic floor muscles) and can easily be shut down by poor posture or breathing habits that mimic abdominal movement, but don't offer the same spinal support. With this change in pressure dynamics and joint mechanics, your lower back is going to hurt more if you haven't figured out how to fire the entire core system. To shift this pattern, switch your posture from leaning back to standing straight, and gently recruit your core with an exhalation as described above. Make sure you aren't clenching all the time or pulling your belly button to your spine (even if you hear this cue in a class!). Use the gentle core contraction to stabilize your body when doing things that appear to hurt your back, like lifting or pushing.

OVERTENSING THE ABS

When people perceive pain or fear oncoming pain, one thing they do at a cellular, subconscious level is brace for impact. Those who have experienced a cesarean birth are notorious for this. The pain of the first few days from a simple cough or a sneeze is seared into your brain, because it's searingly painful. You learn quickly to brace with all movements.

This behavior can be healthy. Bracing for a cough or sneeze as your incision heals makes total sense. Bracing when you carry the dreaded baby-plus-car-seat combo into the doctor's office makes sense, too (even if you know it would be easier to just lift it once into your snap-on stroller . . .). What doesn't make sense is keeping your abs or entire core system tight all the time.

Muscles need length, tension, and a full range of motion to be healthy. Tense muscles are often dysfunctional. They compress things we don't want compressed, like organs, nerves, arteries, or veins. They cause joints to move ineffectively, which leads to impingement or one of the -itis conditions, like bursitis or tendinitis. They will make your fascial system think it's under attack and create a web of tension in your torso.

Many people with fascial tension in their core have a host of symptoms: abdominal pain, indigestion, bladder pain, urinary hesitancy, urinary retention, incontinence, constipation, pelvic organ prolapse, painful intercourse, and back pain. How do you correct this? Stop tensing your body all the time. This simple act goes a long way. You can use a heating pad on your abdomen and give yourself a gentle nightly belly rub with your favorite lotion or oil. Massage lightly and take full breaths. Inhalations with the diaphragm should cause the abdomen to stretch and the pelvic floor to let down. This signals to your nervous system that it can relax; it doesn't need to be hypervigilant and tense when you are at rest.

Consider this: When your pet shows you its belly, this is a sign of respect and trust. When you engage with your belly, you should show yourself the same respect and trust. The intentions in your touch can tell your nervous system to be calm and relax. Conversely, your intentions can reinforce to your body that something is wrong and it needs to remain hypervigilant to protect itself. Accepting yourself and your belly just as they are can be challenging, but letting your abdomen be soft when it's at rest rather than "sucking it in" and hiding it is an important healing step, even as you progress to gently allowing tension again.

DIGESTION-RELATED ABDOMINAL CONSIDERATIONS

Poor management of pressure in the core system can push it in different directions throughout the abdominal cavity and cause issues with digestion. Pressure upward to the stomach and diaphragm can contribute to sensations of reflux or nausea. Downward pressure when lifting a heavy or awkward load can lead to accidental farting, fecal or urinary leakage, or prolapse.

Just as an abdominal massage can reduce constipation, a little bit of core activation can improve bowel movement and stool motility in the colon. This is one reason why you need to be able to activate your abdominal wall. If the skin on your abs looks loose and wrinkly, it's likely that you need to work on activation to stimulate your digestion.

Too much activation can have a "twisting yourself into knots" effect and lead to constipation. This is usually worse if you are a person whose pelvic floor mimics the tension in your abdominal wall. Remember, a Kegel tells the organs *not* to empty. Constant contraction tells your body it's not time to poop, and doing this over and over again can mean your body is not emptying frequently or efficiently. It can also lead to pain with bowel movements or bladder emptying, hemorrhoids, and too much pelvic tension for people who had a perineal tear or episiotomy. If this is you, work on using your breath to help your pelvic organs expand and let down.

LINKING THORACIC SPINE
AND RIBS TO CORE FUNCTION

Every muscle has a spinal level that sends it nerve signals for functioning, which is another reason we think of the core as a system. The abdominal wall gets its nerve signals from the thoracic spine, the section of vertebrae from your shoulders to the spot where your ribs end. Weakness or pain in the abdominal wall can be caused by nerve compression or irritation in the thoracic spine. Improving sensation in your belly means paying attention to posture and movement in your spine and ribs. If you have been having a lot of upper back pain, go back to chapter 5, "Posture," and work on the exercises for your spine and ribs.

The ribs and thoracic spine also connect to core function through muscle attachments. The abdominal and lumbar muscle groups connect the ribs and the thoracic spine to the pelvis. They share a point of origin with the diaphragm, which also works to oppose the difficult-to-treat psoas muscles. Positioning of the thoracic spine and ribs can help you better utilize that deep core system—the diaphragm, abs, pelvic floor, and lumbar groups—for better control. Working this system can reduce that pesky psoas tension.

Nonoptimal positions of the ribs and thoracic spine can present like a high sternum, with a prominent anterior rib cage and a wide infrasternal angle. In this position, your front abdominal wall is lengthened from ribs to pelvis, and separation of the ribs increases, while the distance between the ribs and pelvis in the back decreases. In folks with diastasis recti, this separation of the ribs can contribute to the separation of the right and left rectus abdominis and make it harder for you to support your midline. You are likely to dome or cone with head lifts lying down. This position can also lead to chronic loading of the psoas and constant nonspecific lower back pain. Remember from chapter 4, "Breathing," that this is linked to "inhale up, exhale down" breathing, which is not optimal for the deep core activation necessary to reduce stress urinary incontinence, and to a nervous system that is upregulated because you are holding yourself so rigidly and breathing so shallowly. This is a high-tension position and comes with all the risks of PFM hypertension. If this sounds like you, you need to relax, stretch your lower back, work on back body breathing through positions like child's pose, and restore the transverse abdominis.

The other nonoptimal rib and thoracic position is low tension. It presents as a stuck, rounded upper back, slumped down with shoulders forward. This posture tends to compress the diaphragm down onto the abdominal contents, making it not want to lengthen on the inhale down breath, instead causing a forward and backward belly breath. This pairs with a rounded or tucked-under buttock/pelvis. You may tend to avoid hinging from the hip, instead lengthening the lower back muscles. In these postures, it's hard for you to connect with the glutes because they may be on all the time. The hamstrings will always feel tight. You may have lower back pain from always loading lengthened back muscles. The shoulder blade stabilizers, the lower trapezius and the latissimus dorsi, may not function well with pushing and pulling; you may find yourself holding your breath with every arm task and will likely have neck pain. The core here may fire just fine, but the positioning of the ribs, thoracic, lumbar spine, and pelvis puts a lot of pressure on the pelvic organs and the PFM. They may lock in place and be able to clench, pulling to midline, but not be able to lift. This can lead to increased heaviness/pressure symptoms or prolapse. If this sounds like you, work on training your back, using exercises like bird dog; hinging from the hip; postural openers like open the book (page 114); and strengthening your shoulders. Watch your chronic sitting postures for dropping the ribs down and tucking the buttocks under.

The long-term goal is getting your ribs and torso into a neutral position. From neutral, you can help your core and pelvic floor turn on automatically by breathing correctly when they're needed, without your always having to consciously activate or clench the core. Save that extra tension for movements or load-bearing activities you know are difficult or which trigger pain or symptoms.

HOW TO FIRE UP YOUR BEST CORE

Getting the core to fire appropriately is a crucial aspect of recovery, especially if you need to do a lot of lifting and carrying or want to return to conventional exercise. Practice finding your core with a gentle exhale, preferably with tight lips, and not like a sigh. A core contraction should look and feel like the space between the ribs and pelvis is tightening, with control increasing from the bottom up. This will help the pelvic floor and pelvic organs have the most support. Avoid creating more tension at the rib line and bulging out your lower belly (below the belly button). You should feel a gentle pulling in and up all around the torso, and your bones shouldn't need to shift around to accomplish this. Ruth usually tells her patients to imagine they are making a bed, smoothing the abdominals from pelvis to ribs, sliding in and up, rather than trying to fold the mattress (as in a crunch).

Here are some cues and tips for firing up the core:

* As you exhale, imagine zipping the pubic bone up to the belly button.

- Tell yourself to lift your bladder up higher in your body.
- Imagine you are wrapping your torso in plastic wrap.
- Gently pull the belly away from the waistband of your pants and up.
- Pull your belly button up toward your ribs.
- Pull your abs together in the front.

You should be able to practice this in every position you live in. The key to your success will be to monitor your posture to try to stay neutral, which will in turn increase your ability to hold neutral for longer periods during the day. You should also be able to let the abs go! If you are an overclencher, just turn the abs on and then focus on turning them off. Limit yourself to 5 contractions at a time, or you could rachet up the tension with each rep and find you're unable to relax afterward. If you are overly soft, as signaled by shapeless and easily wrinkled skin over your abdomen, practice activation first and then hold tension for up to 10 seconds, with a goal of 10 reps.

BRACING SUPPORTS

Because we live in a capitalist society and your internet usage has been fed through every possible algorithm to market you "body improvement" products, it's likely that you've seen ads for belly braces, wraps, binders, or shapers. These are all slightly different, but do you really need *any* of them?

It depends on a variety of factors. The hope is that you will retrain your body and learn to use muscle strength rather than rely on a brace forever. However, for folks whose work requires them to stand for prolonged periods or who have only a few weeks of parental leave, a brace might make returning to work possible. If you cannot complete functional tasks like going to work, walking in the grocery store, or doing your laundry due to pain and weakness, then you should try a brace.

Lumbosacral Stabilizing Orthosis (LSO)

A lumbosacral stabilizing orthosis, or LSO, is a medical brace that insurance might pay for if you are working with a PT and you have a qualifying diagnosis, like back pain. This brace wraps around your torso with two Velcro straps and typically has a secondary system that you pull from the back to create an uplifting sensation for your vertebrae. These braces are effective at reducing back pain in folks with poor core activation. You can also purchase one from an online retailer, using funds from a health savings account if you have one, if eligible.

Binders and Shapers

Another type of brace is a binder or shaper, which reduces the size or protrusion of your belly. Because there's money in shaming people for not having a flat stomach, such devices are big. While we want to tell you to kick those patriarchal beauty standards to the curb and embrace the soft round belly that grew a human, we know that's easier said than done. For some, not appearing conventionally "fit" or "attractive" might incur a mental health cost that's more than you can afford. For those whose pregnancy didn't end in parenthood, hiding the shape of your body to avoid unwanted questions might be better for your health. For others, binding is a form of gender-affirming care. You deserve to be your best self, and adaptations to your body shape may be necessary for your mental health and self-esteem. That said, the narratives we hear about our bodies, from ourselves and others, are often untrue. We are all influenced by our perceptions and biases. And no matter what, your body deserves love and acceptance for the way it is right now.

To be clear, binders and shapers do not make your abs stronger. They can also increase downward pressure on the pelvic organs and pelvic floor or upward pressure on the diaphragm and stomach. These are not recommended for people with GERD, hiatal hernia, abdominal hernia, urinary incontinence, or prolapse. One short-term use for binders and shapers is to "reshape" loose skin. This might be particularly helpful to those with an abdominal pannus, which is a large overhanging protrusion of the abdomen that is mostly skin and fat. An abdominal pannus can feel heavy as the day goes on and contribute to the growth of yeast if the underbelly is not kept dry. It can also make it difficult to find postural neutral in standing and can be linked to back pain. If you are not sure if your abdominal pannus is causing your pain or a heavy sensation in your belly, try to lift it up. If your pain or heaviness instantly reduces or resolves, then a brace or supportive garment can be a useful tool until you are able to build up your core strength.

Binding around the core and pelvis can also reduce dysphoria in trans men or other people who prefer a less feminine hip shape. If it's essential to your mental health that you reduce your pelvic and core width, then go for it, with the following considerations:

- Find a compression garment that reduces your pelvic and belly width without overly compressing your central abdomen, which can cause the symptoms we want to avoid. Shorts that compress from the thighs to the ribs are a great way to achieve this.

- We do not recommend binding the abdomen with an Ace wrap, as it is tricky to get the correct amount of compression or to get evenly distributed compression, which can lead to too much pressure on your internal organs.

- A tight belt or sacroiliac joint belt can also pull the pelvic bones closer together to reduce the appearance of wider hips.

Whatever the reason you use a brace, binder, or compression garment, be aware of the length of time you wear them. We do not recommend wearing them to bed, as this can lead to blood vessel and organ compression. Your lymphatic system needs time to drain at night to reduce any swelling in your pelvis and legs, making nighttime compression a bad idea. Daytime compression may be intermittent, alternating four hours maximal compression with a removal period of at least an hour to reduce constriction of the organs and diaphragm. Binding that is too compressive will also reduce rib and diaphragm movement. When the binders are off, practice finding your neutral posture and do some of your other core exercises, and make sure your ribs and diaphragm can expand and you can let your belly down all the way. Wear such a garment to exercise only if you cannot perform the exercise without it or the exercise is too painful without it. Seek medical care if you continue to have pain and symptoms that aren't going away.

CORE EXERCISES

Chin-Tuck Head Lift

Placing a pillow under your head, lie on your back with your knees bent and your arms at your sides. Practice tucking your chin and looking at your knees. With an exhale breath, hover the back of your head off the pillow, without bending it too much. Watch/feel for belly movement. The belly should harden, but not bulge forward, dome, or loaf in appearance. Use your hands on your belly to feel if the upper belly is tighter than the lower belly. Aim for adding lower belly support to "lift the bladder up" to reduce pelvic floor and organ pressure. Work up to 10-second holds; do 10 reps. (You may need the decompression bolstering mentioned in chapter 5 if your ribs are flared.)

Pelvic Brace

Sitting in a chair in anatomical neutral, exhale and activate your lower abdominals and pelvic floor muscles. Envision lifting your bladder up. You should feel all four quadrants of your abdominals activate: right upper, left upper, right lower, and left lower. PFM can assist as well but should not feel heavy. Practice doing a pelvic brace with position changes like getting out of bed, rising up from a chair, or lifting objects. Hold the muscle action for 5 to 10 seconds, and practice being able to sustain the muscle pressure while the diaphragm breathes in and out.

Isometric Obliques

Lie on your back with your knees bent. Perform a pelvic brace and pull one knee up to 90 degrees. Using your opposite hand, press into the thigh of the raised leg. Create counterpressure with both leg and hand until you can feel your upper abs on the arm side and the lower abs on the leg side respond. Hold 5 to 10 seconds. Repeat up to 10 times on either side. This is particularly useful to highlight the external obliques (upper abs) as opposed to the internal obliques (lower abs). Make sure one is not doing more work than the other. Exhale to enhance the pelvic floor contraction either before ("blow before you go") or during ("exhale with exertion") the contraction. Either way, blow up!

Dead Bug Progressions

Lie on your back with your knees bent. Lift your arms up toward the ceiling at shoulder/eye level, with straight elbows. This progression gets its name from the fact that when you are in the starting position, your body resembles a dead bug, with arms stretched up toward the ceiling and legs bent at a right angle above the body, shins facing the ceiling and knees directly above the hips.

1. **Leg raises:** Exhale and brace. Lift one leg up toward the ceiling, bending the knee to create a right angle. Hold. Exhale and lift the second leg into the same bent-knee position. Do not allow your back to arch or your abs to bulge/dome. Hold for 5 to 10 seconds or until you feel yourself losing core control. After the initial exhale to activate, you should be breathing freely. Lower back down with control.

2. **Heel taps:** Bring both legs up into the bent-knee position. Exhale, keeping your knees bent. Tap one heel back down to the floor and return it to the bent position. Alternate legs. Work up to 10 taps per side. Stop if you are losing control of neutral, or bulging or doming.

3. **Arm raises:** Bring both legs up into the bent-knee position. Keeping your knees bent, exhale and raise one arm overhead with a straight elbow. Return to the starting position. Alternate. Stop if you experience shoulder pain or lose control of spinal neutral. Stop if you're unable to control ribcage or core stability. Work up to 10 raises per side with good core and spine control.

4. **Opposite arm and leg:** Combine heel taps and arm raises. When you tap with the right heel, raise the left arm. Reverse and repeat. Stop if/when you lose core control. Stop if there is pain. Work up to 1 minute total.

5. **Straight leg lowering:** Bring both legs up into the bent-knee position. Practice straightening one leg and slowly lowering it to the surface. Pay attention to your core. Stop lowering if you cannot hold anatomic neutral. No arching or tilting! Work up to 10 lowers per side.

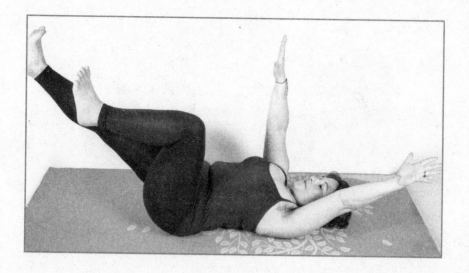

6. **Full dead bug:** Bring both legs up into the bent-knee position. As the left leg extends toward the floor, raise the right arm up overhead. Return to the start position with arms at eye level. Repeat. Work up to 10 times on each side. Remember the goal is good core control during the movement.

Front Planks

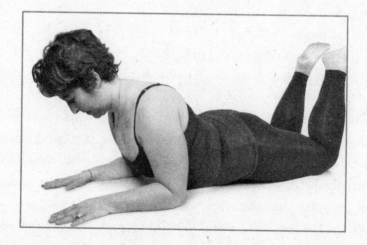

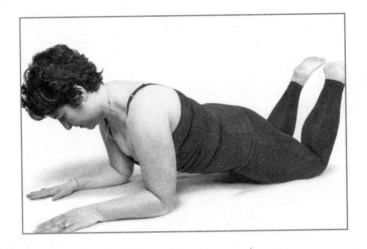

Knees to forearms planks: Lie on your belly. Bend your knees. Prop your-self up on your elbows (see image at bottom of page 205). Look straight ahead and lower your shoulder blades away from your head/neck. Exhale and lift your torso up into a plank (see image above). Keep pressure on your forearms, shoulder blades down, pubic bone connected to ribs for central core support, glutes clenched for a straight pelvis and spine. Do not round the upper back. Breathe! Hold 3 to 5 seconds to start. Repeat up to 5 times. The long-term goal is to build your endurance to 60-second holds.

    Toes to forearms planks: Lie on your belly. Keep your legs straight and turn your toes down to put pressure on the balls of your feet, heels in the air. Prop yourself up on your elbows, palms down. Look straight ahead and lower your shoulder blades away from your head/neck. Ex-hale and lift your torso up into a plank. Keep pressure on your forearms, shoulder blades down, pubic bone connected to ribs for central core support, glutes clenched for a straight pelvis and spine, weight on the toes evenly distributed without turning the feet or ankles out. Do not round the upper back. Breathe! Hold 3 to 5 seconds to start. Repeat up to 5 times. The long-term goal is to build your endurance to 60-second holds.

Toes to hands planks: Lie on your belly. Keep your legs straight and turn your toes down. Place your palms on the floor in front of your shoulders. Look straight ahead and lower your shoulder blades away from your head/neck. Exhale and push your torso up into a plank with straight arms. Keep pressure on your hands. Keep your shoulder blades down, back of the neck long, neck straight, pubic bone connected to ribs for central core support, glutes clenched for a straight pelvis and spine, weight on the toes evenly distributed without turning the feet or ankles out. Do not round the upper back. Breathe! Hold for 3 to 5 seconds to start. Repeat up to five times. The long-term goal is to build endurance to 60-second holds.

Side Planks

Forearm to knee plank: Lie on your side with your knees bent and feet pulled behind you. Turn your lower forearm out so it is perpendicular to your body and your elbow is beneath your shoulder, palm down. Place your upper hand on your ribs or on your pelvis. Keep your neck straight. Push up into a side plank. Head, shoulder, ribs, pelvis, and knees should be in a straight line. Keep the shoulder blade away from ears/neck, glutes activated, pubic bone connected to ribs. Hold 3 to 5 seconds. Stop if you experience shoulder pain. Work up to 60-second holds on each side.

Forearm to heel plank: Lie on your side with your knees straight and legs stacked on top of each other, pressure on the bottom heel. The bottom elbow is bent, elbow beneath shoulder, shoulder blade down, palm down and forearm perpendicular from the body. Place your upper hand on your ribs or on your pelvis. Keep your neck straight. Push up into a side plank. Head, shoulder, ribs, pelvis, and feet should be in a straight line. Keep the shoulder blade away from ears/neck, glutes activated, pubic bone connected to ribs. Hold 3 to 5 seconds. Stop if you experience shoulder pain. Work up to 60-second holds on each side.

Straight arm to heel plank: Lie on your side with your knees straight and legs stacked on top of each other, pressure on the bottom heel. Place your upper hand on your ribs or on your pelvis. Keep your neck straight. Push up into a side plank with a straight bottom arm. Hand beneath shoulder, shoulder blade down, head, shoulder, ribs, pelvis, and feet should be in a straight line. Keep the shoulder blade away from ears/neck, glutes activated, pubic bone connected to ribs. Hold 3 to 5 seconds. Stop if you experience shoulder pain. Work up to 60-second holds on each side.

Bird Dog Progressions

Get on your hands and knees. Find anatomic neutral: straight spine, head in line with body, shoulder blades away from ears, pubic bone gently connected to ribs. Perform a pelvic brace. Hold neutral pelvis and spine posture as much as possible. This is your starting position.

1. **Bird dog arm raises:** From the starting position, blow before you go, then raise one arm in front of you, straight elbow, palm down. Do not tip, tilt, tuck, round, or arch your body. This typically occurs right when your hand leaves the floor. Hold the torso still and keep your core engaged. Hold 3 to 5 seconds. Do 10 reps. Then repeat the exercise on the other side.

2. **Leg extension:** From the starting position, extend one leg behind you, keeping your toes on the floor. Do not tip, tilt, tuck, round, or arch your body. This typically occurs right when your knee leaves the floor. Hold the torso still and keep your core engaged. Hold 3 to 5 seconds. Do 10 reps. Then repeat the exercise on the other side.

3. **Leg raises:** From the starting position, practice lifting a straight leg up toward the ceiling without arching your spine or losing anatomical neutral. Hold 3 to 5 seconds. Do 10 reps. Then repeat the exercise on the other side.

4. **Complete bird dog:** Combine arm raises and leg raises with opposite sides while holding pelvic brace and anatomical neutral. Lift right arm and extend and lift left leg without losing core control. Hold 10 seconds. Repeat the exercise, lifting the left arm and extending and lifting the right leg. Work up to 60 seconds on each side for full core endurance.

CHAPTER 9

The Feet

Like the rest of your body, your feet changed during pregnancy. You might have noticed aching, throbbing, and swelling after a walk. Your toes might have looked like sausages. You might have had foot pain, and you might still have it. You might have noticed that your shoes didn't fit quite right. Maybe your old jogging sneakers aren't fitting or supporting you as well. These complaints are not a surprise when we consider all the ways the feet change with pregnancy. With every pregnancy you carry to the third trimester, you will place more stress on the ligaments and tendons in your foot, causing pronation, a reduced ability to hold the foot rigid, lengthening or widening of the foot (a new shoe size), an increased rotation at the knee, and an increased risk of falls due to a poor sense of proprioception, or where you are in space. Your ankles and feet are essential for stability, balance, and walking.

Getting back to feeling strong in *any* standing or walking activity means that we need to rehabilitate your feet. This can be confusing if your feet do not feel different, but Ruth has rehabilitated more than one person with pelvic organ prolapse or stress incontinence using strategic foot and knee strengthening—really. Remember that your body moves and exists as a system. The tendons that hold up the arch in the foot are also innervated from the same spinal level as the nerves that tell the pelvic floor what to do. A disc or nerve injury in the lumbar spine or sacrum can cause weakness and sensation changes in the feet. There are multiple ways that the feet, pelvic floor, and back are connected. Keeping you upright, supported, and able to move reflexively are part of how they all work together.

ANKLE MOBILITY

The ankle is the joint that connects the foot to the legs at the talus bone, which sits between the two lower leg bones: the fibula and the tibia. The fibula and tibia are the bones that stick out on either side of the ankle. Below the talus is the calcaneus, the heel bone; together these four bones comprise the ankle. Pregnancy changes your range of motion, reducing the amount of dorsiflexion, or backward bending of the foot, which is needed for walking and descending stairs, in particular. Without it, you are likely to twist your foot and turn out or overuse your hip flexors, which can lead to pain in the knee, hip, pelvis, and back.

Ankle Mobility Exercises

Ankle Pumps
Sitting or lying down, point (plantar flex) and flex (dorsiflex) your ankle. Keep it straight. Repeat 10 to 20 times on each side.

Dorsiflexion Mobilization
Standing, place your foot on a chair or a stair. Lean your knee forward in front of your ankle as far as it will go while keeping the heel down. Hold 15 seconds. Repeat 5 to 10 times on each side.

Alternatively, you can do this from half kneeling.

Advanced: Use a resistance band around the front of the ankle to pull the talus back as you lean the knee forward.

Calf Stretch

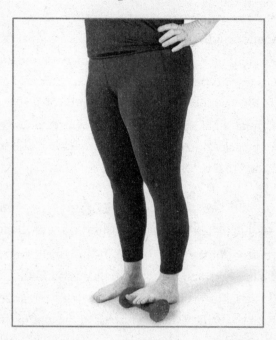

Use a rolled towel, dumbbell, dictionary, or other firm surface 1 to 3 inches in height that you don't mind putting on the floor. Place the ball of your foot—all five bones, don't skip the pinky toe—on top of the surface with your heel on the floor. Check your foot to make sure it's straight (you are probably turned out). Keep your knee straight or locked. Shift your body weight onto that heel and forward until you feel a stretch in your deep calf, and maybe all the way up to your pelvis. The non-stretching leg can be placed on the floor next to the stretching leg. Stepping it backward decreases the stretch. Stepping it forward increases the stretch. Hold 1 to 3 minutes. Repeat 2 to 3 times on each side.

Authors' note: This is the best calf stretch that exists. No other calf stretch has you put your body weight into the heel, which is especially useful for folks with pelvic floor tension to stop the overuse of your hip and pelvis due to loss of ankle mobility.

Lateral Ankle Mobility

From an anatomic neutral standing posture, take a wide stance. Shift your hips to one side and bend that knee. Slowly increase the knee bend and lower your hips toward the floor. Press into the outer heel of the straight leg and look to lift the inner arch of the foot until you feel a stretch on the outer ankle of the straight leg. This is a complex stretch, so you might also feel your groin muscles, knee, or outer hip stretching. Hold 10 to 30 seconds, and repeat 3 to 5 times on each side.

Plantar Fascia Mobility

The plantar fascia is a large, triple-layered, thick connective tissue that protects the bottom of the foot. When it's inflamed, we call it plantar fasciitis, which is a common pregnancy-related condition.

Get on all fours. Turn your toes under so your heels are in the air, but your weight is on the balls of the feet instead of the tops of the feet. Slowly rock back, loading the toes and bottom of the feet. Hold 15 to 30 seconds. Repeat 5 times.

ANKLE STRENGTH

After you've built ankle mobility, you no longer feel like your tendons and fascia are screaming during our mobility exercises, and you can easily move the ankle in all directions, it's time to strengthen. Strengthening will provide you with a stronger foot and ankle to push off from and land on, which can increase walking speed and reduce swelling.

Double Heel Raises

Make sure you are in anatomic neutral standing posture. Push your body weight up onto the balls of your feet, focusing on the big toes; don't roll out. If you can't stop the rollout, try putting a 2- to 4-inch ball between your heels or hold on to a counter and do this in front of a mirror so you can see your feet. Raise your heels up as high as you can and return to the floor. Repeat up to 40 times (the burn will stop you until you gain strength).

Single-Leg Heel Raises

Stand on one leg in pelvic neutral—no hip dropping—and foot neutral—no turnout. Raise up onto the ball of the foot, focusing on keeping your weight over the big toe. Complete 10 to 40 reps. Repeat on the other leg. Doing these without rolling out to the pinky toe, leaning forward, or throwing your body weight around requires a lot of strength. If you are struggling, start with full range of motion and build up to the target reps as you become more proficient. Being good at the single-leg push-off improves athletic performance in those planning to return to regular sports, fitness, or high mileage recreational activity.

Standing Foot Raises

Standing in anatomic neutral, balance your weight on your heels and raise the front of the foot off the ground. Do not lean back. Complete 10 to 20 reps. Do one foot at a time to make it easier.

TOE WORK

The long tendons of the toes help with ankle joint stability, as the muscles themselves are in the lower legs and cross the ankle joint. The shorter toe muscles help with arch stability, as most of them also make up the three layers of the plantar fascia.

Toe work does not have to be complicated to be useful. You may find that these are difficult to do if you have lost mobility, never walk barefoot, wear heels often, always wear rigid shoes, or wear tapered-toed shoes.

Big Toe Extension

Seated or standing, practice lifting just the big toe straight up in the air. Repeat 10 times. Try to keep the other toes relaxed without lifting or scrunching them.

Four Toes Extension

Seated or standing, practice lifting toes 2 through 5 off the floor while keeping the big toe down. Repeat 10 times.

Toe Crunches

Practice curling your toes all together into a towel, like you are bunching the towel between the ball of the foot and the toe pads. Repeat 10 times.

Advanced: Practice picking up other things, like marbles.

Advanced 2: Do this standing.

THE ARCH OF THE FOOT

Once your foot feels like it's moving normally again and you've regained basic strength in the larger muscles, it's time to work on how those areas interact. The main thing is making sure you can hold the shape of the medial arch of the foot instead of letting it fall flat. These movements are called supination (arch increases) and pronation (arch decreases). You need both when you hit the ground and push off from it.

Check Your Arch

Standing in anatomical neutral, ensure the inside border of your foot is not touching the floor. Put pressure on the outer heel and the ball of the big toe to help. Practice flattening and lifting the arch without lifting the toes or the heel from the ground.

Challenge: Do this with a resistance band wrapped around both feet and push the arch up without rolling the ankle.

Challenge 2: Do this while taking steps forward and backward.

Arch Supports

Some of you will find that you don't do a great job of holding up your arches, no matter how much you practice. This can be worse with fatigue or the amount of time you need to be on your feet for work. You might need arch supports in your shoes during the day, which will help reduce rotation and strain in the knee. If you've had a knee ligament or meniscus injury, you might find your knee hurts more with certain footwear.

Many shoes come with built-in arch supports; these are marketed as stability shoes. You can also buy over-the-counter versions. Consider arch supports if you experience more pain or fatigue in your lower body joints, including your feet, knees, hips, or low back, after long periods of standing, or if your job includes a lot of standing and walking. Look for shoes with more cushion if you work on hard surfaces or just have to stand without moving for a long time, like cashier work. They're like a built-in anti-fatigue mat.

Athletic Shoe Choices

Arch support either as an orthotic or a rigid shoe is controversial in sports and fitness wear. The main issue is that the foot needs to rotate and pronate with push-off and landing. It's a way that the body is efficient with movement. The bottom of your foot is like a trampoline, just like the pelvic floor. You can't just make something rigid that is supposed to bounce and expect it to function properly. Some other part of the body that relies on that flexibility (in this case, your knees) will be more prone to injury without the proper functioning of this trampoline.

Sneakers come in a variety of styles for different needs and foot shapes. Normal walking involves rocking from the heel to the ball of the foot and pushing off the big toe, and any pair that you own should pass this test. Moving easily from your heel to the balls of your feet and pushing off from your toes with force is required for landing and loading. Look for a shoe with enough room in the toe box for you to be able to separate your toes, crunch them, and lift them to some degree. In the long run, shoes with a tight toe box increase the possibility of bunions, which are painful and can impact how you move. (We both have square Hobbit feet and don't enjoy the feel of a tight toe box. We also both prefer function over fashion, and thankfully there are more fashionable, functional shoes on the market than ever.)

Stability shoes, those with a lot of support, tend to work for folks who don't have reliable ligament, tendon, or joint support in their feet due to injury or disease, such as recurrent sprains, rheumatoid arthritis, diabetes, or hypermobility syndromes. Such shoes help you keep some arch support for push-off without allowing the arch to fully collapse. Neutral shoes are a good middle option. These have basic arch supports without any changes to the structure of the shoe. High mobility shoes or free-form style shoes allow maximal mobility, which allows you the greatest awareness of your joints and of the ground beneath you.

Make sure you are choosing a shoe based on your needs for an activity, taking into account how long you expect to be doing the activity. The salespeople at a good athletic shoe store can be a tremendous help. Maybe you need a stability shoe with a high top for hiking, a neutral running shoe, and a free-form shoe for CrossFit. Weightlifting shoes tend to have a small heel lift without arch support, which locks the heel in place and can overcome a tight ankle that limits the depth of your squats or your hip angle. Engage a salesperson if you are looking to streamline your shoes for your budget and cannot buy three pairs. There are many neutral cross-training shoes that may be a good fit.

There is no perfect shoe, but you can make a good match between what your body needs for the task you want to do. Think about getting rid of shoes that you wore during your pregnancy, especially if they are for a specific task or sport. They are broken in for your pregnant body, which was moving differently. You don't have that body anymore.

FITNESS AND SPORTS

Before diving into your favorite sports, make sure you have gotten your feet ready for landing and pushing off. This challenges the load and power of the foot, along with your legs. These movements will also rely on your hip and back mobility. If you notice problems, make sure you run through chapter 7, "The Lumbopelvic System," as well as this chapter.

Single-Leg Balance

With your standing knee straight and your trunk in anatomic neutral, lift the opposite foot off the ground, keeping the thigh parallel to the standing leg and the knee bent. You can keep the toe of your lifted foot gently on the ground for more support to start, or use two fingers on a wall, chair, or counter to help you balance. Hold this pose for 60 seconds, then do the same on the other side.

Knee Drive

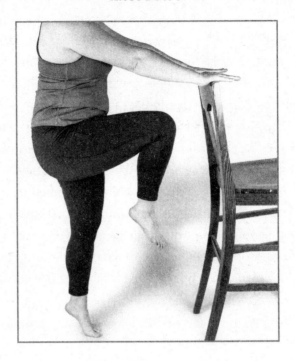

Put one foot flat on a step. Drive the opposite knee up as high as you can with a gentle forward trunk lean. Lower back down with a straight spine, allowing the stabilizing knee to bend.

Do this up to 20 times to ensure you have the quad and hamstring strength to control your leg. If you notice the knee turning in, check and make sure your arch is not dropping and that you have enough hip control. Repeat on the opposite side.

Modifications: Holding a chair or wall will increase your stability as you build leg and trunk control, as shown above. You can also keep the stable leg straight to focus on driving the moving knee upward. For an added challenge, add a heel lift in your standing leg to the knee drive. The taller the stair or the step is, the harder this will be.

Step-Downs

From a stair or step, face as if you are going down. Allow the knee to go forward of the ankle and step down slowly. This is a great way to ensure you have functional dorsiflexion for hiking and going downhill. This is also a great way to strengthen your quads for knee stability. Start with a short step and increase the height for a challenge. Complete at least 10 reps on each leg.

Authors' Note: About ten years ago, trainers and therapists stopped letting people get their knees in front of their ankles during squats and lunges. It's unclear why, and this cue could be relevant if you were training for a specific style of squat in a competition. Also, allowing your knee to go in front of your ankle increases the load in your knee, particularly the meniscus and ACL, so if you have injuries in these areas, you might not want to do this frequently or with a high load. However, this cue took on a life of its own, and now people think they should *never* allow their knee in front of their ankle. This is markedly untrue. You would never be able to walk downstairs or downhill if you always followed this advice. Allowing the knee in front of the ankle when appropriate decreases the load on the hips and low back and reduces the likelihood of hip injury and pain. Train for what you need to do with your body. Be careful of fitness trends.

Single-Leg Dead-Lift Swing-Throughs

Holding a weight in each hand, bend one knee and lift the leg (see image at top of page 222). Send the other leg back behind you with a neutral spine (don't arch the back), leaning forward as far as you can without losing your balance (see image at bottom of page 222). Hold your balance this way for 10 seconds, then pull the knee forward and through until you are standing up tall again with your hip and knee at 90 degrees. Repeat this cycle. It will challenge your single-leg stability and core strength at the same time. Stand next to a wall if you need balance support. Repeat up to 10 times with each leg.

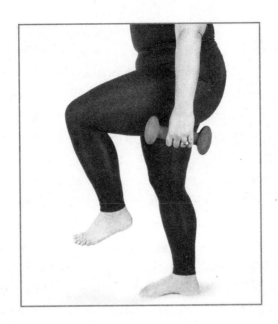

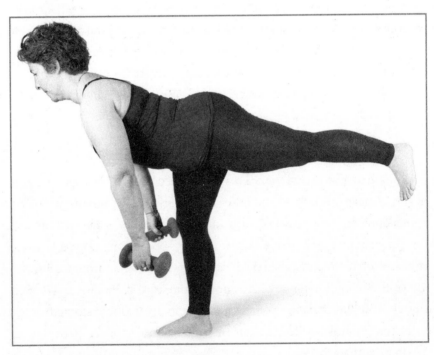

Side Jumps and Hops

Practice jumping a little out to the side. Do this barefoot. Look at your arch and knee when you land. The arch should be up and the knee should be a little bent and in line with or slightly in front of the ankle. Start with double foot jumps and progress to single-leg hops. Wear stability shoes to support your arch if needed.

As you get comfortable, practice larger hops and slide the moving leg behind you. These are commonly called ski jumps or slaloms.

Be light on your feet. Think about how soft and quiet you can be in the landing. See if you can initially land on the ball and arch of the foot without immediately dropping to the heel.

Plyometrics

Repeated fast and forceful activities where you land on your forefoot are typically called plyometrics, also known as high intensity interval training (HIIT) or aerobics. These activities all rely on the two properties of feet we talked about: being able to hold your arch to create a lever that pushes you up in the air, and being able to use your mobility to land on your foot as if it were a trampoline, providing energy and allowing you to rebound into the next jump, hop, skip, etc.

Plyometrics are high-level exercises. They will require you to have baseline strength in the other areas of your body and a good handle on your posture, breathing, and pelvic floor. We want all your trampolines firing together so that you can be successful, which means reducing urinary leakage, prolapse, and pain upon landing and repetition. Think about your plyometrics in terms of your foot. Are you landing on the ball of your foot? Are you landing lightly? Do you have strength to propel yourself off the floor? Is your ankle stable when you land? If not, and if you are having any of the above symptoms, add dumbbells or other weights to any of the strength exercises we've discussed and get stronger in your feet before you get frustrated about leaking on your landing. It's not always your pelvic floor's fault when things don't go to plan.

CHAPTER 10

Putting It All Together

THE PISTON SCIENCE METHOD:
POSTURE, BREATHING, ABS, AND PELVIC FLOOR

Everyone wants to know the special sauce for physical recovery. How do two people doing the same exercises have different outcomes? How does one person doing core and pelvic floor strengthening manage to stay dry and well-supported while the next person has prolapse and leaks? Reintegration of the core by activating the breathing system is the key. As Julie Wiebe, PT, puts it, "It's where the puzzle comes together." The person who has done the work to pattern their movements, letting the system function together, will have an easier time than the person fighting it or winging it.

Wiebe realized that the exhalation breath is the pump of the deep core system, teaching the Piston Science approach of pelvic floor integration to other PFPTs who wondered why the use of Kegels alone wasn't curing patients of their symptoms. Piston Science is named after the up-and-down pistonlike action of the diaphragm and pelvic floor in the abdominal cavity. Other folks might call this method of using breath for deep core activation the canister, the pop can, or the connection breath. In chapter 6, we called this the pressure management system. All these names describe coordination of the breath with reflexive muscle activation to reduce leaking and the risk of prolapse. This is the way the system is designed, and your goal is to intentionally integrate the teamwork of the deep muscle systems by practicing movements repetitively to restore automatic or reflexive activation.

Imagine a balloon to picture what this integration looks like. On a balloon, it's easy to see how increased tension in one area causes a pressure reaction elsewhere. Imagine squeezing it in one place and seeing it bulge in another. The system *should* reflexively respond to that pressure by snapping back like a rubber band that has been released from a stretch. This is most easily driven by coordinating the posture, diaphragm, abs, and pelvic floor. Throughout a normal breathing cycle, we see the interaction and counterbalance of the different parts of the system all the time: inhalation loads the system; it responds with a stretch when the diaphragm descends; pressure builds; on the exhalation, the ribs, abs, and pelvic floor recoil; and the diaphragm lifts, taking the abs and pelvic floor with it. This is the "blow up!"

Here are a few reminders about breath and posture: Breathe with your diaphragm, allowing it to descend and your lower ribs to expand when you inhale and recoil on your exhale. Stand in readiness for movement, with shoulders and arms relaxed, head in line with your body, leaning slightly forward. Don't turn the abs and pelvic floor on in readiness. Keep them soft so they can respond to changes in posture or breath. These cues can be enough to allow your abs and pelvic floor to respond to movement automatically instead of feeling like you have to lock them down.

This might feel counterintuitive and even scary, but these simple cues reduce symptoms of leakage in many of Ruth's clients. Leaning forward activates the pelvic floor for better bladder control, and breathing signals your deep system to respond. Less cueing to squeeze and lift will result in less overthinking and will improve your ability to move in a way that supports your organs and spine without symptoms.

Easy Cues to Improve System Automation

- Blow before you go.
- Exhale with exertion.
- Do a quick exhale on landing a single jump.
- Release belly/core tension: Relax those abs!
- Lean forward and shift your weight onto your toes using your entire torso, not just slinging your pelvis forward.
- Don't hold your breath.
- Inhale into the lower ribs, expanding them like an umbrella.
- Stand with your legs wider apart than usual.
- Change your eye position: Look slightly down at the horizon about twenty feet away.
- Add rotation to your favorite movements to practice not gripping your ribs or upper abdominals.

Listen to your body and trust it to give you feedback on the best ways to train. If you notice that one of the above cues helps you to leak less or reduces pain, use it. Instead of adding pressure or contraction at this stage, spend time just moving and breathing and see what brings you toward your goals of less leakage, bulging, and pain.

Becoming hyperfocused on one body part (ahem, you chasers of the flat belly) means overtraining for tension instead of reflexivity. Over time, you will train your body to become less responsive. A "more is more" mentality or a fear of pain or symptoms can lead to overclenching for simple movements. You don't need to use 100 percent effort for every movement, even in a workout. Gentle intentional muscle activation might be useful to reduce leaks while you are still building foundational strength, or when you are moving or bouncing a load that is too heavy or one that may potentially cause leaking (we cannot always manage our loads and reduce the weight we manipulate in the real world). Just remember to match tension between the abs and the pelvic floor—if the abs overpower the pelvic floor, there will be downward pressure. Continue to work toward moving and breathing in a way that the system is responding on its own.

Once you free yourself from excess tension in your abs and pelvic floor during recreational and functional movement, you can learn to let each system fire reflexively. We hope that freedom will reinstate your willingness to find joy and playfulness in your movement. How do you move, run, jump, or dance when you add play, joy, and fun into the mix? Does this result in fewer symptoms and less pain?

PLANNING
AN EXERCISE SESSION

When you're ready to return to traditional exercise, a plan can help you to train safely. Start slow and small. Pick three days per week when you know you can work out. Speak with your partner or family members about giving you time to exercise. If you work outside the home and have reliable transportation, try to exercise when you are already out of the house. Once you go home, there may be too many calls on your time to prioritize working out.

If you work at home or prefer working out at home, maybe tie your workouts to something else in your routine, such as fitting in a 30-minute session right after the baby is fed. Or perhaps your workout can be included in the time your baby spends at day care or with another caregiver. If you have a supportive partner or family member available, coordinate with them to give you 30 minutes of sacred time when you are unavailable. If you tend to jump in and help if you hear the baby crying, consider listening to music or using noise-canceling headphones.

FITT:
FREQUENCY, INTENSITY, TIME, TYPE

Once you have a plan for when and where you'll work out, use the principles of FITT (frequency, intensity, time, and type) to return to exercise intentionally and safely.

FITT Principles for Exercise Planning

PRINCIPLE	RECOMMENDATION	OTHER CONSIDERATIONS	TECH SUPPORT/ PRO TIPS
Frequency	• Start with three to five days per week, with a rest and recovery day between sessions.	• If you feel sore or heavy, add another rest day or scale the intensity down. • Exercise only if you've gotten 6+ hours of sleep. • Recover back to baseline between sessions.	• Fitness watches to monitor heart rate variability and body battery and recovery needs based on percentage heart rate can help determine how frequently to exercise.
Intensity	• Cardio: 40 to 60 percent of max heart rate to start, slowly building up to 85 percent. • Resistance: 8 to 12 reps of a weight that starts to feel challenging at the end.	• Begin with low to moderate intensity, like walking or stationary bike. • Set a goal of successfully repeating your routine 10 to 30 minutes five days a week. • Consistency is queen.	• Percentage of max heart rate range calculation: (220 − your age) × .4; repeat and multiply by .6
Time	• 10-minute sessions, adding 5 minutes each time you successfully recover to baseline.	• Add time only if you successfully recover to baseline. • Don't increase time and intensity in the same session.	• Begin with a longer session if you practiced the same exercise consistently until the end of pregnancy.

FITT Principles for Exercise Planning

PRINCIPLE	RECOMMENDATION	OTHER CONSIDERATIONS	TECH SUPPORT/ PRO TIPS
Type	• Anything considered exercise, from aerobics to Zumba!	• Walking is the number one exercise recommendation. • Nature is healing. • Walk with friends. • If you can, walk without carrying or pushing the baby (at least sometimes).	• Hills and stairs are the resistance training of walking. Flat terrain and levels are much easier to start with.

FIIT Recommendations for Specific Types of Exercise

WEIGHT TRAINING

Train your large muscle groups (biceps, triceps, deltoids, pectorals, back, quads, glutes, and calves) two to three days per week. The weights you use should be enough that you feel resistance but can still breathe and keep your ribs over your pelvis. Holding your breath, leaning back, catching the weight against your hips, or being unable to stabilize your torso mean your weights are too heavy. Use a lower weight if you have pain at any scars or increased symptoms of heaviness, bulging, leakage, or pain. If you can throw the weight through space without any effort, it's not heavy enough. You should be tired at the end of 10 to 12 repetitions.

CARDIO

Cardio or aerobic training is work for the purpose of attaining and sustaining 40 to 85 percent of your heart rate max, calculated as 220 minus your age. For those in childbearing years, this is likely between 80 and 160 beats per minute.

The goal of this training is endurance, activity tolerance, and heart and lung conditioning. If you have been sedentary, begin with 5- to 10-minute sessions three times a week and gradually build to 30-minute sessions with no or very light added load once you have established consistent practice. If you remain symptom free with this added time, consider adding intensity through speed, resistance, or hills. This will increase your working heart rate. At higher heart rates, you may need more rest days to recover your function, and this work can increase the risk of muscle pain, fatigue, leakage, or prolapse. Let yourself recover before repeating the exercise, and reduce time or intensity if you find your symptoms are worsening. Resist the urge to give in to the "more is more" mentality. Use your plan and goals to motivate you through every step of your healing process.

FLEXIBILITY

We recommend flexibility training once or twice a week, which can include yoga, Pilates, or stretching. If you plan to stretch, do it after cardio or resistance training. Stretching before an activity is linked to weakness in the tendons and a reduction in your ability to generate maximal force and power in your muscles, which can cause injury or pain. Remember that your postpartum pelvis and abdominals are already overstretched, so don't go for broke. Make sure you're stable in your foundational posture and can breathe in the stretched position. Hold each stretch steadily, with no bouncing, for 15 to 60 seconds. Stop right away if anything hurts. Pain may be a warning signal to your body that you are putting too much pressure on tissue or simply an indication that you are moving in ways you haven't in a while. Ease into your end ranges and decide if pain is information or a warning sign.

HIIT

High intensity interval training, or HIIT, combines cardio and resistance training with impact movement and is often considered a full body workout. These exercises often require strength, baseline cardiovascular fitness, the ability to move a load/resistance with speed and control, and the ability to tolerate impact. Examples include cardio kickboxing, step aerobics, circuit training, home body workouts like MommaStrong, and elements of CrossFit. HIIT may not require much equipment and online classes can be done on your own time, both of which make it an attractive option for a return to exercise. However, because HIIT programs focus on elements of power and speed, getting back at it may require modifications to load your core without symptoms. Do fewer reps, move at your own speed, reduce or avoid impact, and make modifications if necessary. For instance, you might find mountain climbers to be hard to sustain while breathing and holding a partial plank. Scaling this exercise down may require putting your hands on a bench, slowing down the movement, or completing it in a 1-2 pattern, then resting with your knees on the floor. Scaling down burpees would reduce the entire movement to its parts: stand, bend, hands on floor, step back one leg at a time, lower to the floor in a way you can control, push up, step back in, stand up with arms up without the jump. Many classes and online programs offer postpartum-specific and/or lower impact workouts, so start there and make sure you have good form and no increased pain or symptoms before increasing time, speed, impact, and intensity.

WHAT IS THE GOAL OF THE EXERCISE?

Your postpartum return to exercise can look however you want it to. But make sure you know what goal(s) you're trying to accomplish. Here are some examples:

- I want to move my body.
- I want to play with my kids.
- I want to rejoin my fitness community.

- I want to get stronger.
- I want to become more flexible.
- I want to reduce my risks for heart disease.
- I want to have strong and healthy bones.
- I want to reduce my markers for anxiety and depression.
- I want to reduce pain.
- I want to have more energy.

You may want to write down your goals and plan in a journal or notes app to make it concrete and help hold yourself accountable. You'll notice the absence of any goals related to weight—this is not that book. We acknowledge that there are complex social pressures around body shape and weight, and you may negatively compare your pre- and postpartum body. But that all underlines why you should set exercise goals related to function and feeling to crowd out those other voices and guide you toward a return to movement that's in line with the work you've done to recover and heal.

Here are two sample goals and plans:

Ruth wants to exercise because it makes her happy and helps her sleep well. She also gets a real thrill from doing headstands or being able to do any paddle sport at any time without prep work. She is going to plan her exercises around developing a strong core and upper body for her chosen sports, and then she is going to prioritize exercises that make her happy, usually including sprints, weightlifting, or recreational sports. She is going to plan to do arm exercises two to three days a week, focusing on multiple movements and using medium weights that she can do 10—but not 20—repetitions of, in 1 to 3 sets or rounds. She can mix her core workouts into her arm days and use the other two days a week to do some kind of cardio that makes her happy, like taking an exercise class or running sprints down her road while her neighbors wonder what is wrong with her.

Courtney wants to exercise because it helps her mental health and reduces her recurring lower back and TFL pain. Her favorite activities are swimming, cross-country skiing, and walking, so she'll do those whenever she can fit them in and the weather permits. If she can't get outside for a while, she will substitute with an online walking or dance cardio workout. She likes lifting weights because it feels good and supports her swimming and skiing, but she knows she has better form and safety when she works with a coach, so she plans a weekly session with a trainer at the gym who can show her exercises for her whole body. She tries to do one additional session at home each week to practice what she learned with her trainer and might sneak in a little mat (living room rug) core work when there's time. She also subscribes to an online HIIT program designed for pregnant and postpartum people and tries to do a daily 5-to-15-minute workout from there.

ORDER OF OPERATIONS

If you like to mix up your exercise sessions to include distinct categories, plan your session with your goal activity first. For instance, if you want to train for cardio to eventually run a 5K, do not start with stretching or weight training. You will want to save your energy for the main training task, so go on that run first. If you want to gain muscle mass, then begin with resistance training and cool down with a light cardio activity. Limit your secondary activities until you have regained a baseline for pushing yourself in multiple categories.

MODIFY BEFORE YOU QUIT

If postpartum symptoms or injury are getting the best of you, figure out how to modify your activity level rather than quitting. In resistance training, reduce the number of exercises, reps, or sets you do, or reduce the amount of weight you lift. Avoid painful lifts and continue pain-free lifts. For cardio training, reduce time, intensity, or frequency. Reduce hills, drag (e.g., wind, pushing a stroller, riding a bike with a trailer on it), exercise-equipment levels, or resistance. Slow down. Combine low pace cardio with workout pace cardio to get your preferred training time. Layer in rehabilitation exercises (chapters 4 through 9) to restore stability, range of motion, and coordination, if you sense any loss in those areas.

PROGRESSING TO SINGLE-LEG EXERCISES

Single-leg exercises are often a litmus test for sport readiness. If you have a pelvic health therapist, they will probably ask you to do this so they can give you personalized recommendations on how to improve your form. If you don't have a therapist or coach, record yourself doing exercises and watch your posture and breathing. Most sports require some degree of single-limb stance time, as well as the ability to push off in one or multiple directions. You'll know you're ready for single-leg exercises if you can do the following without musculoskeletal pain, scar pain, incontinence, heaviness, bulging, or pressure in your pelvic floor or core:

- Squat
- Bridge
- Side plank

- Front plank
- Heel raises
- Dead bug
- Bird dog
- Single-leg balance

Exercises to Advance Single-Leg Tolerance, Strength, and Impact

Authors' Note: Integration breathing for lunges and squats is *Inhale on the way down, exhale on the way up, or BLOW before you get up.*

Reasoning: The pelvic floor is lengthening into a squat and shortening coming out of one. Appropriate diaphragm cues help the rest of your deep core system activate without creating too much intra-abdominal pressure or overloading the pelvic floor.

Lunges

1. **Front lunge:** From standing anatomic neutral, step one leg forward. Keeping neutral posture, lower the back leg as low as you can go without pain or loss of balance. The back heel should lift, allowing pelvic neutral. The front leg should be flat in the foot and bent at the knee. Inhale with the lowering, exhale with pushing back up to start. Return to start. Switch legs.

   a. **Progression:** Step ahead enough to lower the back leg to the ground, with the front leg bent at 90 degrees.

   b. **Progression:** Start from half kneeling with one leg in front of the body, foot on the ground, 90/90 bends in the hip/knee. The back leg is bent with pressure on the knee, toes turned down. Hands are on hips or crossed over the chest. Press up to tall lunge: the feet should not have moved, front foot flat with partial knee bend, back leg heel raised, weight on toes, pelvis neutral. Slowly lower back down to half kneeling, or a partial range that you control with ease.

c. **Progression:** Build strength by holding dumbbells or a kettlebell with the movement, 8 to 12 reps each side.

d. **Progression:** Practice rowing with pulleys or resistance bands in the lunge position. This is a great place to practice eye gaze, forward lean of the trunk, and breathing with movement to develop integration habits.

2. **Rotation lunge:** Tall lunge position: front knee bent, foot flat, pelvis neutral, weight on ball of the foot/toes on back leg, knee slightly bent, body leaning forward slightly. Practice rotating the pelvis and trunk in the direction of the front bent knee. The pelvis should rotate into the front leg. Try squeezing the thighs together if you are having trouble.

a. **Progression:** Add a resistance band or pulley cable to the rotation. Resistance in front: With arms out in front of the body at chest level and elbows straight, hold the band in clasped hands. Resistance at your side: If your left leg is in front, the resistance is on your right side. Rotate into the front leg, against the resistance. The straight elbows/clasped hands should stay straight, and the movement should come from the core and pelvis. Repeat 10 times on each side.

b. **Pallof press:** Stand in tall lunge. Use a resistance band or pulley in both hands with elbows bent at chest height. The band should be at your side, away from the front of the leg. Step away from the band until you have full tension and mild to moderate resistance while holding the band at your chest. Hold a neutral lunge position with the band in your clasped hands. Push the band/pulley straight ahead at chest level. Resist the rotation of the band (it will want to pull you toward the wall/anchor). Push and pull the band toward and away from your body holding neutral tall lunge position. Do 10 reps. Turn around and face the other direction to switch sides.

3. **Side lunge:** Standing in anatomic neutral, bend one ankle/knee/hip as far as you can and slide the other leg straight out to the side with your foot flat on the ground. The bending side should stay in neutral, with ankle, knee, and hip in alignment without deviating to the side. The sliding leg should have a foot that faces straight ahead, a straight knee, and an arch that doesn't collapse or touch the floor. Step or slide back to start. Repeat 10 times each side.

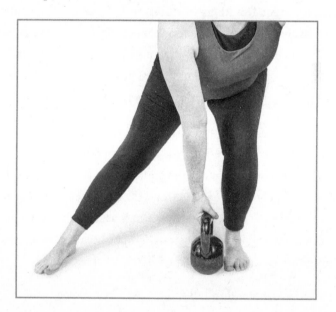

a. **Progression:** Complete with a medicine ball held at the chest, or dumbbells in your hands to increase leg strength.

b. **Progression:** Step out to the side as far as you can, trying to touch the floor in front of you, holding a neutral front leg. Return to start.

c. **Progression:** Step out to the side with dumbbells or kettlebell. Try to touch the dumbbells to the floor next to the front leg. Stand and return to start.

d. **Progression:** In the deepest part of the lunge, punch/rotate into the front/bent leg 5 to 10 reps.

Squats

1. **Chair squats:** From a chair, practice a squat. Legs are apart, hands on hips, crossed over the chest, or out straight in front of the body. Lean forward, shifting weight onto the feet/legs. Press up to stand with a neutral spine.

   a. **Progression:** Hold a medicine ball, plate weight, or kettlebell against your chest as you complete the stand. Repeat 10 times.

   b. **Progression:** At the top of the stand, squat back down as slowly as possible and hold 10 seconds before totally sitting back down.

   c. **Progression:** At the depth of the squat without sitting, practice rotating your trunk and punching your arms at a diagonal, 5 to 10 punches with each arm.

2. **Single-leg chair squats:** Sit at the edge of a chair. Place one foot/leg out in front of the body, and one leg bent at knee and ankle nearer to the chair. Lean forward and shift your weight until you load the leg nearest the chair with minimal to no weight on the front leg. Push up to stand. Repeat 10 times on both sides.

   a. **Progression:** Hold a medicine ball, plate weight, or kettlebell against your chest as you complete the stand, keeping the front leg fully off the ground in front of you. Repeat 10 times.

b. **Progression:** At the top of the stand, squat back down as slowly as possible and hold 10 seconds before totally sitting back down.

c. **Progression:** Sit to stand on a single leg from progressively lower surfaces for deeper core and leg strength.

3. **Single-leg squats:** From anatomic neutral standing, hands on hips, across your chest, or straight out in front of the body at chest level, hinge at the hips with a straight spine, bending at hip, knee, and ankle. Descend into a controlled, neutral squat. Kick one leg out in front, putting weight only on the back leg. Press back up to start. Repeat 10 times on each leg.

a. **Progression:** Go right into a single-leg squat. Stand in anatomic neutral. Take the pressure off one leg by either bending it behind you or holding it straight in front of you off the floor. Squat as low as you can on the weight-bearing leg while maintaining anatomic neutral in your spine and pelvis. Straighten to return to stand. Switch to the other leg and repeat.

Dead Lifts

1. **Regular dead lift:** Standing in anatomic neutral or slightly wider, hinge at the hips while holding a neutral spine. Drop your buttocks toward the ground without allowing your knees to pass in front of your ankles. As you progress, you should be able to touch the floor with your fingertips. Repeat 10 times.

a. **Note:** Weighted dead lifts are NOT the same as unweighted dead lifts. Weighted can be easier.

2. **Single-leg dead lift:** Standing in anatomic neutral, lift one leg behind you with a bent knee. Hinge at the hips while holding a neutral spine,

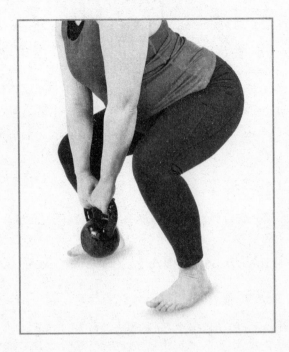

so that you lean over the front toes as far as possible. Send the back leg back as far as possible while holding neutral spine and pelvis position. Stand back up tall and pull the back leg forward. Repeat 10 times per side.

IMPACT READINESS CHECKLIST

Are you returning to impact sports? This might include running, ball sports, or HIIT exercise. You should be able to do the following first:

- ☐ Walk for 30 minutes.
- ☐ Balance on one leg 60 seconds without support.
- ☐ Jog in place 1 minute.

- ☐ Leap forward 10 times on each leg by running about 10 feet then jumping into the air, extending one leg in front of you and one leg behind you.
- ☐ Hop in place with legs together 10 times.
- ☐ Jump forward with both feet 10 times.
- ☐ Hop side to side with legs together, 10 repetitions to either side.

STRENGTH READINESS CHECKLIST

Are you strong enough to start playing a sport again? See if you can do the following:

- ☐ 30 repetitions of single-leg heel raises on each leg with good arch control
- ☐ Single-leg squat, 20 repetitions on each leg
- ☐ 20 repetitions of a single-leg bridge with straight leg raise
- ☐ 20 repetitions of single-leg sit-to-stand
- ☐ 20 repetitions of the straight leg raise in abduction
- ☐ Pelvic floor muscle 10-second holds, 10 each in standing and lunge positions
- ☐ Single-leg dead lift, 10 repetitions on each leg
- ☐ Forearm to toes plank: 30 to 60 seconds
- ☐ Side plank forearm to heels: 30 to 60 seconds on both sides
- ☐ Bird dog: 60 seconds on both sides
- ☐ Dead bug, 20 repetitions on each side

YOU SHALL NOT PASS: CONTRAINDICATIONS AND PRECAUTIONS FOR RETURN TO SPORTS AND EXERCISE

If you are having the following symptoms, speak with your physician before starting any exercise routine or sports:

- Vaginal/genital bleeding: current, not associated with known and normal menstrual cycle; passing large clots or bleeding that begins after exercise

- Abdominal pain

- Hypertension: blood pressure above 200 mm Hg for the top number (systolic) and above 110 mm Hg for the bottom number (diastolic)

- Aneurysms in the brain

- Chest pain

- Frequent joint dislocations

- Dehydration

- Calf pain/swelling or known blood clots in the legs, deep vein thrombosis

- Poor response to exercise, including an inability to regulate body temperature, an inability to get your heart rate back down after 30 minutes along with palpitations, a sensation of fainting or loss of consciousness, headaches that begin with exercise and do not go away after 30 minutes, severe fatigue

- RED-S: relative energy deficiency in sport (formerly known as female athlete triad syndrome), caused by excess energy expenditure with inadequate replacement. Can include poor/inadequate nutrition, poor/inadequate sleep, excessive exercise/energy expenditure, and increased daily demands. Can cause infertility, bone mineral density loss, loss of menstrual cycle, changes in cardiovascular health, compromised immunity, changes in metabolism, pelvic floor dysfunction, and impacts on psychological well-being.

INTEGRATION EXERCISES TO DETERMINE PREPAREDNESS FOR SPORTS

Dumbbells/Kettlebells

Free weights can be many things. The main thing here is to move with intention. Most weight movements are asking you to hold neutral, which requires paying attention to your core system to resist the urge to lean back or to the side or bear down to get the weight to move. Try to figure out how to move the weight through space with the least amount of extra body movement. Keep the effort low at first just to see how it feels. As you gain confidence, you should be able to increase your weight. For now, your goal is 8 to 12 reps. Increase your sets as your endurance improves. Increase the complexity of the movements as your stability and confidence improve.

The best way to avoid a pressure injury is to breathe with the exertion of the movement. Usually this is when the weight moves away from the body. The more speed and power you use for your lifts, the more stability and more "piston" coordination you will need. Remember what your pressure injuries are: diastasis recti, pelvic organ prolapse, incontinence during exercise, hemorrhoids, hernia, or herniated discs in the spine. If you have had more than one of these injuries, be extra careful that you aren't prioritizing speed and weight in your lifts. You need stability before all else to remain injury-free.

Exercise Ball

This is a large ball, usually about 55 to 75 centimeters in diameter, that you can use with any workout. They are great rehabilitation tools because they can help people adapt their programs without having to quit entirely. One of Ruth's favorite uses for an exercise ball is to teach a body how to bounce again. Sit on the ball (with good shoes or bare feet), practice finding neutral, then practice bouncing. Start with a small amplitude bounce. Let go and feel how your core and pelvic floor are turning on automatically with impact. Feel how you might be holding yourself rigid and need to reduce some body tension. Prioritize an exhale on the impact of the bounce if you are having prolapse, heaviness, or leakage symptoms.

Exercise balls are also a tool for upper body weightlifting if you notice that you don't feel comfortable doing standing lifts just yet. They can help you to be more body aware in case you tend to lean to the side or slouch. Try biceps curls, overhead press, and forward punch for starters. The exercise ball can also be used from kneeling to help return to planks and weight bearing without asking a ton of your core right out of the gate. Think walkouts to straight arm planks, arm and leg bird dogs over the ball, upper back flys, or kneeling over the ball for support if your cesarean birth scar is still healing and positioning yourself on your hands and knees still feels unsupported.

Body Weight Exercises

You need no equipment for most body weight exercises, such as mat-based yoga and Pilates. The goal is stability, or finding neutral, then reaching, bending, or twisting from neutral. Each movement or hold in neutral builds postural stability over time. They can also be tiring, requiring rest breaks so that you don't do too much at once. Typical body weight exercises are planks, bridges, squats, and lunges. Your goal is to be able to hold them with good, pain-free form first, then make sure you can breathe easily while you hold them, and finally move in and out of them faster.

HIIT and Jumping

This is the final piece of pelvic health recovery, because jumping assumes baseline strength, joint stability, good exercise capacity, and the ability to generate and respond to power. The end game is to be soft on landing without losing joint control. Everything about HIIT is about being light, using momentum, absorbing impact into the next part of the exercise, and changing pace with control. With Piston Science breathing, we want you to stay rubbery, lock nothing, and breathe to remind your pelvic floor to stay mobile.

Start with double leg jumps with your legs together. Gently jump forward or off a one-inch step. Make sure you can do this without symptoms. Practice jumping to the side with both legs together. As you get better at this, practice bounding, or taking small forward leaps where you must land on one leg. You can do this in a star pattern: forward, side, back. Repeat. Focus on the softness. How far can you move with a soft landing and heels elevated? The shock absorption part of the foot is the ball of the foot and arch. See if there's a difference between wearing your favorite athletic shoe and being barefoot. As your system responds more reflexively, you won't have to think about the separate parts as often, you will feel springy, and you will be able to jump farther and longer as your endurance builds.

The Jump Rope Test

The jump rope test is designed to measure your capacity for regular or repetitive jumping. You should start with supportive footwear (or barefoot if you prefer) in a clear area. Get onto the balls of your feet as if ready to jump. Knees are bent, hips are bent, spine is stacked but pliable, slight lean forward, chin down. Practice jumping up and down in place. Stop if/when you feel a leak, increased prolapse/pelvic pressure, or any bowel/bladder urgency. See how softly you can jump. Can you bring in the element of play, but still have control in the movement? Remember your cues: lean forward; keep your eyes on the horizon 20 feet in front of you; make sure you get a full inhale *down*. As you get better, see if you can jump on one leg. Add the rope when you feel ready to get the timing right. If you feel your symptoms, check in with yourself. Did you lose form? Did you hit the ground too hard? Did you lose your breathing? Are you just tired and that's all the system can do at one time? With regular practice, the different parts of the system should start to bounce without loss of control. If you have a prolapse, you might need a pessary in to feel successful with this.

Part 3

. . .

RETURN TO SPORT

Greetings, Postpartum Humans! Welcome to part 3, where we detail safely getting back into your favorite types of exercise. This is for anyone who wants to *return* to one of the exercises listed: yoga, Pilates, running, kettlebell, or CrossFit, or general sports.

If you're interested in a certain type of exercise but have never done it before, note that we'll be using specific terminology that assumes prior knowledge of the activity. We will not get into the nitty-gritty of each movement, so some familiarity will be helpful. However, if you're starting to work with an instructor, you can use these chapters as a guideline to do so safely.

You do not have to read these chapters if they do not interest you.

CHAPTER 11

Planning for Sports and Fitness

WHEN TO GET BACK TO YOUR USUAL SPORT OR FITNESS ROUTINE

Here's the rub: No one knows. We are serious. The American College of Obstetricians and Gynecologists' position is that no research has reported severe outcomes from starting exercise postpartum. That is, there is not enough evidence warning against it, and there are plenty of benefits for your total health. This includes exercise for people with diastasis recti, tears, and surgical scars.

Our hope is that after reading part 2 you are empowered with information about your strength, healing process, and the benchmarks to look for to know when you're ready for more intense activities. Remember not to exercise or push yourself if you have warning signs of poor healing or poor general health, listed in chapter 10. If that's you, speak with someone on your medical team to understand if, when, and how to exercise.

HOW TO GET STARTED

If you are skilled in exercise regression and modification, you can start a light version of your favorite fitness activity. The key is to know when to progress, when to regress, and how to modify if you are having symptoms, regardless of when you start or how many weeks you are postpartum. If you're watching videos, use a mirror or video yourself to check your form. Limit your reps to what you can do with good form. You'll fatigue quickly at first, so honor and respect that as you regain strength and conditioning.

If this is all feeling daunting, look for an instructor with pregnancy and postpartum athleticism certification or a pelvic health therapist who can give guidelines to your coach or trainer, as they don't all have this knowledge. It's offered as a continuing education credit and not included in general teacher training programs (eye roll).

The runner-up is the instructor who is open to talking to you before or after class, hearing your concerns, and offering modifications. Having an in-person coach who understands and supports working at your own pace is critical for safe training and mental health. If possible, avoid any instructor dismissive of postpartum modifications or those unwilling to make suggestions when you have symptoms.

Everyone can benefit from the exercises we described in part 2, and they're particularly beneficial for those of you who don't know where to start and/or who have symptoms of poor body integration. You get to decide how to use them:

1. Proceed with your chosen activity while doing part 2 to build baseline fitness.
2. Wait to start part 3 until you've cleared the checklist from part 2.

Need more input? Courtney Wyckoff, founder of MommaStrong, a functional fitness program for pregnant and postpartum people, says you should be able to have a conversation in the language of functional fitness. That is, are you able to coordinate your breath and pelvic floor muscles (PFM) so you're not overloading with pressure during dynamic movement? Do your head, torso, legs, and feet feel connected, like they're all part of the same human? Are you listening to your body in terms of the big three—rest, hydration, and nutrition—and feeling filled up, rather than depleted, when you work out?

If so, keep going. If not, go back to part 2 (particularly chapter 10) and continue to build your functional baseline.

WHEN TO MODIFY

Modify your normal routine if or when you experience leaking or incontinence, bladder or bowel urgency, pressure, or prolapse. Talk to your doctor if you have vaginal/genital bleeding that occurs consistently after exercise. Back off when you're extremely tired or have had fewer than six hours of sleep. Take days off when sick or recovering from illness.

ARE YOU HAVING PELVIC HEALTH SYMPTOMS BUT STILL REALLY WANT TO EXERCISE?

Here are some thinking points in your decision-making. Does the social component of the class encourage you to maintain a regular practice? Are the people you exercise with or around *your* people? Being in community and having a sense of belonging are such an integral part of a person's support structure and sense of self that this may be a vital part of your total health and wellness. If your exercise group is part of your social support network, staying engaged can better serve you than stopping due to symptoms. Consider ways to attend class that allow you to participate—that is to say, wear a pad, dark workout pants, or a stability brace—and add focus to your form. Notice when you experience symptoms—is it right away, or does it get worse with fatigue? Can you do half the class, half the reps, or no/low weight? What modifications allow you to stay and keep coming back? How can you build consistency by showing up with a little work now so you can get back to the big stuff without injury later?

GENERAL FITNESS CONSIDERATIONS

Here are some general fitness considerations to keep an eye on:

1. **How often are you exercising?** You want to allow time for your muscles to recover between sessions (which requires good rest, hydration, and nutrition). We recommend one day between moderate exercise sessions and two days between heavy exercise ones. If you are working light, you can exercise every day.

2. **How long are your fitness routines?** Sixty to ninety minutes may be too long due to the cardiovascular and musculoskeletal changes from pregnancy and birth (which require more recovery days). Try 10 to 30 minutes to start. If your classes are 60 minutes, slow down in the last half or change your general pacing so you don't use all your energy and muscle strength in the first 30 minutes.

3. **What is your exercise motivation?** Are you trying to beat your body into submission for a weight on the scale or a pants size as quickly as possible? As we've said before, this is not that book. With these goals, you're more likely to ignore the signals your body is giving you about control and coordination. This can lead to fatigue, irritability, chronic pain, and issues with pelvic floor pain and dysfunction, and it may even affect lactation. Working in a low-calorie intake, high-output deficit does not give your body what it needs for recovery. If you experienced postpartum circumstances such as scars, delayed healing, hemorrhage, or a child who was in the NICU, you may find you need to eat even *more* to support tissue health and healing. As we've mentioned before, make sure your "why" is more than a number (weight or size) and is something you can enjoy and celebrate every time you show up.

4. **How hard are you working?** Showing up is the goal right now, and modifications are the pathway to meeting it. You're not training for a personal record or a new skill! Challenge yourself to be honest about your needs and your form. This work will help you get PRs down the line, but right now, your job is to work smarter, not harder. As other trainers put it, "slow is fast" right now.

5. **How is your form?** Have you done the rehab work to rebuild coordination, breathing, posture, and muscle strength? Every single coach we interviewed wanted to make sure their clients had prepared to return

to sport by doing precisely that. Flip back to part 2 to review that work. You can do those exercises and your sport in a modified way if you have the time and inclination. You might find you use those techniques to stay injury-free in the long term, well beyond what most people consider "postpartum."

6. **Go to class!** Working through part 2 at home might feel impossible, and your exercise class might be the only shred of alone time that you can carve out. Get there! Use parts 2 and 3 for reference to get ideas for modification and to understand your body's pain and fatigue cues. Sneak in some of the rehab exercises as a warm-up or cooldown. Make it work for you.

7. **Please consult with your physician about your readiness to return to activity,** especially if you had a postpartum stroke, a heart condition, a hypertensive emergency such as preeclampsia or eclampsia, or a major issue with any other organ. When you do speak with your physician, be specific about what exercise means to you. How high are you allowed to get your heart rate? Are there warning signs you should be aware of? Is there a weightlifting limit? Take care of yourself and adhere strictly to their parameters.

CHAPTER 12

Yoga

For many, yoga is a practice of foundational physical and mental health. To the typical Western practitioner, yoga offers strength, flexibility, breath work, balance, coordination, and meditation. Classical practices, based on the Yoga Sutras of Patañjali, are intended to be a full eight-limbed way of life, or Ashtanga yoga (*ashtanga* literally means eight limbs). This includes self-practices called *yamas*, or principles of how to behave in the world including nonviolence (*ahimsa*), truthfulness (*satya*), non-stealing (*asteya*), abstinence (*brahmacharya*), and non-hoarding (*aparigraha*). *Niyamas*, or practices of self-discipline, include cleanliness (*saucha*), contentment (*santosha*), heat (*tapas*), self-knowledge (*svadhyaya*), and full surrender to the divine (*ishvara pranidhana*). The more physical practices of yoga include postures (*asanas*), breathing (*pranayama*), concentration (*dharana*), withdrawal of the senses (*pratyahara*), and meditation (*dhyana*). Practicing these seven limbs leads you to the eighth and final path, enlightenment (*samadhi*).

Yoga comes in a variety of styles and intensity levels. Depending on what your practice looked like before and during pregnancy, returning to yoga might require a shift in mindset. Postpartum is a great time to deepen your practice in breath work and meditation, which is linked to a reduction in postpartum depression. A reasonable schedule is one where you can regularly come to your mat with the intention of expanding your practice in one of the eight limbs for 10 minutes, five days a week.

According to Brianna Bedigian, a yoga teacher and author, "Yoga is a practice of peace, and I believe you can practice yoga in any body you have as long as you're honoring where your body is at that day, that moment. You aren't going after the pose as the gold standard [but] rather, honoring what your body needs." Bedigian's twenty-plus years on the mat enable her to be a better parent by practicing meditation and breath work.

YOGA FOR STRESS REDUCTION

Five to ten minutes each day of lying down with head and knees supported while breathing deeply can reduce stress, which in turn promotes healing and can restore nervous system regulation, says Bedigian. Dustienne Miller, PT, MS, WCS, CYT, who utilizes yoga with her physical therapy patients, agrees. When it comes to postpartum yoga, the practice could look different in this season of life. With goals of being mindful, breathing, and noticing sensation, this practice could entail connecting with breath while lying in your bed on days when you are too exhausted for a more physical practice.

Tension-related dysfunction can occur when we hold ourselves chronically tight, ironically to create a feeling of safety. Creating what feels like a "safe vessel" actually contributes to chronic stress and nervous system dysregulation. If you struggle to release tension or to allow movement and breath into your poses, Bedigian recommends Yin or Restorative yoga. These styles of yoga can activate your parasympathetic nervous system (rest, digest, recover, and arousal systems) by holding poses for an extended period to give you time to settle there. Any practice that reassures your ventral vagal system that you're safe—supported poses, singing, laughing, humming, breathing in sync with a trusted person—can allow you to release tension, she says.

MOUNTAIN POSE
FOR YOUR RETURN TO PRACTICE

Before you hop right into a class, try mountain pose (*tadasana*) at home. Mountain pose is a lovely place to practice finding optimal standing posture after proprioception has been altered during pregnancy. This supports the musculoskeletal relationship of the diaphragm and pelvic floor, enhancing the activation of the abdominal wall, spinal muscles, and hip muscles. If you experience leaking or incontinence, practice shifting your weight forward and back in mountain, relaxing your pelvic floor in each position. Keep your pelvic floor relaxed—there's no need for *mula bandha* (root lock, essentially a Kegel) in mountain pose. Build up your tolerance for time once you feel like you've mastered the basics.

Steps and Considerations
for Mountain Pose

Place your feet hip distance apart, taking a moment to stack your bones from the ankles up.

Lift your breastbone and allow the shoulders to gently fall back and the palms to fall open.

Imagine that there is a string attached to the crown of your head gently being pulled to the sky, lengthening your entire frame upward.

Now begin to move your awareness around the body:

Notice the right hand vs. the left hand, the right hip and the left hip, the belly front to back, the rib cage from side to side. Is one side tighter than the other?

How are you holding the bowl of the pelvis? Are you gripping? Where is your tailbone in space? Does one hip feel tighter than the other? Are you holding a Kegel? Are you bearing down?

What is the stomach doing? Do you feel settled? Are your abs working overtime?

Reset the pose. Stack the bones, lift the chest, let the string pull the crown upward, lengthening the entire kinetic chain.

Add in the breath:

Notice your breath on both its inhale and its exhale. Where does the air go? Is it shallow? Is it deep? Is one side breathing more than the other?

Can you do a 360 breath (ribs move, diaphragm drops, belly moves)?

To automatically deepen your breath, begin with the exhale. Exhale all the air out, then inhale:

Where does the air go? Do the ribs move? Does the back move? Does the breath drop straight down? Where is the pressure of the breath moving in your body?

If you feel constant tension in the pelvic floor and/or pressure going down with your breath, these point to the possibility of pelvic floor dysfunction. Go back to the pelvic floor exercises focusing on relaxation in chapter 6.

RETURNING TO YOGA CLASS

Consider a beginner class, even if you were previously in a more advanced level. Styles of yoga such as Restorative, Yin, or Hatha yoga are supportive and slow enough to give your body time to get used to the pose, breathe, relax, and open into it. The gentler pace and intensity will give you the space to explore the sensations of each pose and build strength. Transitions are slower in these styles of practice, and you should not have to worry about rushing to get to the next pose. Often, instructors have more time to proactively offer modifications to make poses more accessible and comfortable in this style class.

Noticing Sensation

Returning to a practice including *asanas* in a flow requires mindfully noticing sensation. A pose may feel accessible, but the transition to the next pose, the timing, or the breathing may not. Miller and Bedigian recommend exploring your sensation and fluidity during transitions such as rolling over and standing from a seated position (from the floor or a chair) before progressing to a flow class. While rolling over or getting off the floor, ask yourself:

- Do your movements feel restricted?
- Is your fascia (connective tissue) moving smoothly?
- Do you leak during the transitions?
- Do you have more core or pelvic floor heaviness after the transition?

Being able to engage your deep abs (pelvic brace) and understanding how abdominal separation or core weakness has changed your body will help you progress in active yoga styles (like power, flow, or vinyasa practice). Bedigian advises that these styles of yoga include transitions and movements that may create too much abdominal pressure, exacerbating core and pelvic health conditions. For example, in sun salutations, students are cued to move from a forward bend to standing while inhaling (most movement practices use an exhale here). Actively coordinating the deep stabilizing system, including breath, core, pelvic floor, and the movement transition, may prove challenging or feel symptomatic. Mindfulness, awareness, and modification of the poses and transitions may be required as you heal. Prioritizing the breath during these transitions can help activate the abdominal wall and pelvic floor without creating enough pressure to cause symptoms. Remember that research has already told us the core fatigues more quickly in the first year postpartum. Give yourself grace with this information and don't try to correct months of body composition change all in one mat session. Promise yourself to stay curious about your body every time you come to your mat. Work hard to quiet self-comparisons and criticisms. Honor even the days when your progressions feel slow or absent. Every time you come to your mat is an opportunity for non-harming (*ahimsa*), contentment (*santosha*), self-knowledge (*svadhyaya*), and full surrender to the divine (*ishvara pranidhana*) in your postpartum journey.

Flow and Vinyasa

Transitioning through a flow should be approached slowly and mindfully as it includes multiple braced inhales. Hold each pose for long enough to explore your sensations and notice any pain, sharpness, or pressure, using these questions from Bedigian as a guide:

- Does this pose create any pain or pressure? If so, notice where and back off or stop entirely.

- How is your breath? Are you:
  - breathing?
  - able to observe the inhale and exhale?
  - aware of where the air is going?
  - able to deepen the breath?
- Are you holding tension in muscles that do not need to be involved:
  - grasping with hands?
  - tightening face and jaw?
  - clenching pelvic floor?
  - gripping with stomach?
- How do your left side and right side differ:
  - right hand versus left hand?
  - right hip versus left hip?
  - right foot versus left foot?

You can learn a lot from noticing what your body doesn't feel able to do. "With yoga in particular, it's worth it to say, 'Well, why?' I can't engage, I can't twist, if I open my groin everything feels like it's falling out. A lot of powerful information comes through not being able to do something," says Bedigian. "Take that in, then practice in a way that supports your body."

Downward-facing dog (*adho mukha svanasana*) and high (*phalakasana*) and low plank (*chaturanga dandasana*) are poses that you'll find in many styles of yoga. Preparation for down dog and plank can begin with hands placed on a wall, table, or countertop. The closer you get to the floor, the greater the strength requirements in your arms, core, and spine. Progressive loading builds strength and helps protect the body from injury, says Bedigian.

When you're ready, try downward-facing dog on the floor. Begin in tabletop, warming up through a few cat/cow spinal movements, then transition with an exhale, stepping back one leg at a time, and lifting your bottom into the air. Check in with your tailbone. Can you move it in this pose, or does it feel stuck? Can you wag it side to side? Untuck your bottom if it feels winked or tucked under. Can you create length in your spine? Are you able to both push into and rest into your hands to support your spine?

To transition into and out of downward-facing dog or plank, use your knees instead of your toes. Normally you'd transition from downward dog to low lunge, but it's easier to return to hands and knees, *then* position into low lunge. Getting into downward-facing dog from baby cobra (*bhujangasana*), sphinx pose (*salamba bhujangasana*), or upward-facing dog (*urdhva mukha svanasana*) is more accessible if you push back to your knees and then lift your bottom instead of doing it all in one breath or one transition. Until you are used to regular transitions with support, skip cues to hop or jump back into downward dog or plank.

As you regain strength, Miller recommends replacing upward-facing dog with sphinx pose. In sphinx, the stomach, legs, feet, forearms, and hands (palms down) rest on the floor. Press down into the floor with the forearms, hands, and feet while pulling the elbows back to shine the chest forward and open the heart. In this supported, active posture you can achieve a backbend without deeply stretching the abdominal wall. A cesarean birth scar needs to fully close before tolerating this position and stretch. Upward-facing dog is a stretch on the anterior body. Due to this area already being weak, thin, and stretched from pregnancy, be mindful of whether you feel supported by your fascia or whether things feel like they're falling out. Bedigian asks, "Can you hold yourself together and open your heart?" If not, add a gentle PFM (pelvic floor muscles) contraction with a zip-up of the lower abdominals. Back pain or a feeling like you're bending in half is another clue that you aren't reflexively activating your core. This may mean taking a break from the pose, or simply approaching it with curious awareness. For those with fully closed cesarean scars, sphinx with a slow progression to upward-facing dog and other extensions may improve scar tissue mobility and reduce fascial tension on the bladder and uterus.

Plank requires full-body strength and the ability to sustain a pelvic brace. Be sure that your deep internal stabilization system of breath, core, and pelvic floor are communicating and engaged, but not on lock-down. Once you can do that, try stepping back into a plank from tabletop. Engagement is the goal, *not* having a perfectly straight line from your head to your toes. Lift your bottom as needed, and stop right away if you feel discomfort, a falling-out sensation, or pain. This is a challenging place to find the balance between core and pelvic floor tension while still breathing. Comfortably holding a plank for 10 to 20 seconds is a good indicator that you're ready to mindfully rejoin a flow-based class.

Check your standing posture in a mirror. You are (hopefully) mindfully reteaching your system how to find optimal standing alignment with a long and tall spine. Watch for common patterns like dropping your belly out or forward, overarching your back, or shifting your ribs behind your pelvis. This is what Miller calls a "nonoptimal load transfer." Training your body to stack uses the core more efficiently, creating a more optimal load transfer. This position improves management of thoracic, abdominal, and pelvic pressures, which can decrease many postpartum symptoms.

In standing work, two-legged postures like mountain, warriors I and II (*virabhadrasana* I and II), and hip hinges like chair pose (*utkatasana*) while focusing on pulling your femurs (hip bones) backward can build postural strength. You may find it easier to transition to a single-leg balance posture by starting from mountain pose each time. As you gain control, you can begin to move to a single-leg balance from chair, warrior I and II, and triangle (*trikonasana*). Higher-capacity single-leg postures, like warrior III (*virabhadrasana* III), dancer (*natarajasana*), and eagle (*garudasana*), will demand a lot of stability throughout your body and system integration. Exploring these postures can help you discover one-sided weakness and work on your intrinsic foot and arch support, which you know helps your deep core system activate. If you feel these poses and transitions are easy, balanced side to side, and are places you can find peace with a hold, you can progress to hops/jumps in your vinyasa flows.

Inversions can be healing and instructive for your pelvic floor. A gentle bridge (*setu bandha sarvangasana*) and/or a bridge with a bolster while breathing can reduce pressure on the pelvic floor and reduce symptoms of pelvic organ prolapse. Use a chair, bolster, or wall to support you for higher-level inversions like legs up the wall/waterfall pose (*viparita karani*) and shoulder stand/supported shoulder stand (*sarvangasana/ salamba sarvangasana*). Inversions should not make you have pain, pressure, heaviness, leaking, or a sensation of prolapse. Make sure the ones you try are in line with your capacity.

Ruth once treated a postpartum human who was complaining of the dreaded queef. She was having vaginal wind during her home vinyasa practice. It was due to mild vaginal prolapse, mostly present after overdoing it (being the sole caregiver for a tiny human is very tiring), pooping, or at the end of the day. Inversion poses in yoga were the worst. The embarrassment was keeping her from returning to her community practice. Going through a typical vinyasa, Ruth gave her the same cues she is giving you here: check your posture for "extremes," stay in the gray area, and breathe intentionally during the held poses and in the transitions. If you feel heavy, sigh and exhale to release thoracic and abdominal pressure. Don't clench anything on purpose in a pose unless doing so relieves pain. Focus on gentle stacking. For this person, that made all her yoga poses accessible without the "noise," except shoulder stand. Going through shoulder stand, piece by piece, Ruth realized she was locking her throat, holding her breath, and throwing her body into the air without appropriate back strength and core support. Working through the progression of legs up the wall, waterfall pose single to double leg, bridging double to single leg, and progressive core strength in bird dog and boat pose (*paripurna navasana*), she was able to move into a modified version of shoulder stand without dread or unwanted noise.

Returning to heavy ab loading postures requires practice with less difficult poses and slight modifications until you are ready for the full pose. These include *chaturanga dandasana*, boat pose, full plank for vinyasa transitions, crow pose (*bakasana*), or any other arm balance inversions. *Chaturanga dandasana* can be modified with the knees, chest, chin approach to the floor. For boat pose, lean on a wall or chair and lift only one limb at a time. Start with bent knees and progress to straight knees as you learn to hold your core without pelvic floor heaviness or core bulging. Practice crow pose with your hands on the floor and legs resting on a bolster while progressively leaning into your arms.

CONSIDERATIONS FOR MODIFICATION

PFM and *Mula Bandha*

We have already taught you that a constant Kegel is not in your best interests for long-term PFM health. This is not common knowledge (yet!). Some yoga teachers will say, "We are going to focus on the pelvic floor today." While there are teachers that understand this as a complex system, due to a lack of centralized yoga licensing and limited standards for anatomy and physiology, a session with equilibrium between tension and lengthening is not guaranteed. When a teacher focuses on pelvic floor strength only, it can lead to cueing *mula bandha* with *uddiyana bandha* (lower ab engagement) for most, if not all, poses. "Working with the *bandhas* can be a beautiful part of practice as long as engagement is balanced by release. In many yoga classes we are cued to lift and hold *bandhas*, creating a pelvic brace for extended periods of time. This pattern of constant bracing without balance can lead to unnecessary tension," Bedigian says. Remember our discussion about constant pelvic floor tension in chapter 6, and how it can lead to the exact symptoms you may be trying to reduce. If you know you already have symptoms of pelvic floor hypertension—constipation, painful intercourse, constant need to urinate, or urinary incontinence—skip these cues. If you complete a class heavy in *mula bandha* (we know some of us just want to follow class cues) and have symptoms afterward, go into some hip openers with breath to help release the pelvic floor. Ruth often recommends seated or reclined bound angle/butterfly pose (*baddha konasana*), wide angle pose standing or seated while exploring trunk movement side to side or forward bending, happy baby, and the yoga squat (*malasana*) as pelvic floor openers.

Hypermobility

If you experience hypermobility in your joints, take care not to lock your knees in standing poses or arch your spine in downward dog or standing poses. (In downward dog, do your elbow creases face forward? Can you put your hands flat on the floor with your knees locked? These are signs of hypermobility.) Adding a gentle bend to the knees and checking and repositioning your elbows are easy fixes. Avoid pushing yourself to the end or locked range of every pose. Often, hypermobile people put a lot of pressure on their ligaments and joints rather than using their muscles, but pushing into end range of poses like pigeon can make SI joint pain or SPD pain worse. Build stability and symmetry in poses like low lunge and extended side angle pose before progressing to more involved poses, like pigeon or triangle. Where your muscle strength is limited, and it's too easy to lock out, use blocks to support hand positioning or bolsters to reduce the pressure. Hypermobile folks are more likely to feel the pain after the movement is complete or while they are transitioning out of a deep pose.

"Yoga is about the inherent balance between strength and flexibility," Bedigian says. "It straddles the line between tension and relaxation, effort and ease. Give yourself some grace, take some time, explore your body's capacity with curiosity. Finding your equilibrium as you return to and gradually intensify your practice will make yoga a supportive and empowering part of your healing process."

CHAPTER 13

Pilates

Pilates, when taught well and practiced thoughtfully, can be a highly effective way to reeducate your postpartum body and prepare it for other forms of exercise, or you can do it for the enjoyment of the practice itself. Pilates can improve the quality of postpartum sleep, reduce symptoms of depression and anxiety and feelings of fatigue, and increase energy.

If you practiced Pilates before and during pregnancy, you may associate it with core flexion—exercises involving raising your head off the ground while lying down—and exercises involving both legs simultaneously. In your postpartum return, you'll want to gradually build strength and stability through a progression from lying on your back (supine) and working one bent leg at a time all the way back to the full expression of each exercise. The reasoning for this is to reduce intra-abdominal pressure (IAP) on the core (especially if you are recovering from a cesarean birth) and lessen the lengthening effect of crunch style exercising on the pelvic floor. This is particularly necessary for those still rehabilitating from perineal tears or avulsion of the pelvic floor.

Coordinating breath and movement is one of the primary objectives of Pilates practice. Effective breathing requires mobility in the torso, which can be limited when we're holding one posture for a long time, as when we're working at a computer or feeding a baby. Pilates instructor and coauthor of the *Pilates Workbook for Pregnancy* Michael King recommends finding time for some full body movement, such as taking a short dance break during the day, to encourage mobility. Being able to coordinate the breath and pelvic floor, as we discussed in chapter 6, is a prerequisite to resuming your practice.

SUPINE PILATES EXERCISES

Amanda Olson, DPT, PRPC, a physical therapist, a Stott Pilates instructor, and the president and chief clinical officer of Intimate Rose, a pelvic wand and dilator company, emphasizes the modifications available for the postpartum period. She recommends building a progression of exercise from movements lying down on your back, side, or front, to standing and balancing exercises, and finally to more dynamic movements such as rolling.

Olson recommends beginning with modified supine exercises such as the Hundred and the Series of Five. These are typically performed in core flexion and use single- or double-leg movements.

* Lie on your back, with head flat on the mat and feet to the mat, knees bent.

* Inhale, relaxing and expanding your pelvic floor. Exhale, gently activating your core and pelvic floor. You can envision a 360-degree hug from your core that would result in your belly pulling away from the waistband of your jeans. Alternatively, imagine wrapping your torso in plastic wrap. The goal of this pre-movement contraction is to ensure that you have 360 degrees of core support and that you are not overpowering your pelvic floor and creating a downward pressure. (See chapter 8, "The Core," to review.)

* Holding your form, lift one foot off the mat, keeping the knee bent. Replace the foot on the mat.

* Inhale, exhale, activate your core, and repeat on the other side.

Tune into feelings of pain or fatigue. Your core, which has recently been through a whole lot of stretching and change, is likely to tire easily. It's typical in Pilates to perform a certain number of repetitions. However, this makes it more difficult to maintain stability and the tension appropriate to the exercise, so embrace practicing your movements with attention to form rather than counting. Quality, not quantity! Don't push it—stop when your body tells you to. Regular practice is what will lead to an improvement in how long you can go and how many reps you can do, with good form. Form and coordination of the body is the goal.

The next step is to introduce core flexion:

* Lie on your back, with head flat on the mat and knees bent.

- Inhale and relax, exhale, activate your core, and lift your head off the mat.

- March one leg, keeping the knee bent, and replace your foot and head on the mat.

- Repeat on the other side.

Again, pay attention to pain or fatigue. Make sure you can maintain stability in your core and that the core flexion isn't causing leaking, pelvic floor pressure, or cesarean birth scar pain.

Once you can consistently perform the marching movement with added core flexion, without rapidly fatiguing or leaking, the next step is to add a "long lever" movement of the leg, rather than marching. Olson suggests using a Theraband to increase stability:

- Lie on your back, with head flat on the mat, one knee bent and one leg extended long, with a Theraband looped around the back of the knee or the foot of the extended leg.

- Inhale, relax. Exhale, activate your core, and lift your head off the mat.

- Holding the ends of the Theraband, lift the extended leg and lower it fully to the mat.

- Unloop the Theraband and repeat on the other side.

- From here, progress to 4 leg lifts before switching to the other side.

Take the time to rebuild muscle strength, increase endurance, and ensure stability at each step, which could take several weeks or even a few months. Listen to your body and use any pain or increased symptoms as a sign to regress or decrease repetitions.

SIDE-LYING PILATES EXERCISES

Side-lying exercises, such as the Sidekick Series, are inherently more stable than exercises performed on your back. You may recall this is the gravity neutral position for pelvic floor activation (one of the easiest). It may be more accessible than lying face upward for people with lower back pain. Be on the alert for pubic bone pain or sacroiliac joint pain with side leg lifts, as too much abduction can strain these joints. Start with hovering or a tiny lift of less than an inch rather than a large range of motion. Work with small movements that are not painful—a good rule of thumb for all exercise, if we haven't emphasized that enough.

Still having pain? Head back to chapter 7, "The Lumbopelvic System," and work through those exercises to build stability in your pelvic ring. Fatigability of your glutes and core may be the barrier to the side-lying series. Consider bending your knees if this feels more comfortable than working with legs extended long. Remember to keep control, form, and coordination as your primary goals. Do fewer reps or shorten the time if you are losing these in your practice. Still having pain? A visit to a pelvic health therapist might be warranted.

If you have access to a Reformer (a machine used in Pilates), Olson recommends it as a helpful tool in your practice. It provides stability and proprioceptive input, which can give you neurological feelings of safety. Proprioception is an internal knowing of where you are in space. Feeling uncoordinated or having poor balance are symptoms of poor proprioception. The Reformer can allow you to focus on your breath and coordination sooner in the process than mat Pilates alone. It also allows you to control load to an appropriate level, handy while you're progressing. The Reformer reduces pressure on the central abs, which is more comfortable for those of you with a cesarean birth scar.

PRONE PILATES EXERCISES

To progress to front-lying (prone) exercises such as Swimming, begin by just lifting the head off the mat, coordinated with an exhale and gentle core activation. If that doesn't feel good in your lower back, assist yourself by pressing into the ground with your hands as you lift. Once the head lift feels stable and consistent, lift and lower one arm 8 to 10 times, then the other, then each leg in turn. From there, lift and lower the right arm and left leg together, set them down, then repeat with the opposite arm and leg, for 8 to 10 repetitions. After working through this progression for six to eight weeks (or more!), progress to the full fluttery swimming movements of the exercise.

STANDING PILATES EXERCISES

Standing exercises are often performed in the Pilates stance, a heels together, toes apart turnout. However, your stance may naturally be more turned out than it was before pregnancy. Try a variety of postures for standing exercises, including feet parallel, turned out, and turned in.

Olson offers the following progression to the push-up, an example of a standing Pilates exercise. These elements can be practiced as separate pieces.

- Begin kneeling or half kneeling, and practice a gentle forward spinal roll.

- Practice the upper-body elements of a push-up. Focus on controlling and connecting through your shoulder blades. Progress from wall push-ups to countertop, bench, a kneeling plank, and a kneeling plank with shallow dips.

- Increase the depth of your knee push-up until you can lower gently to the floor and press all the way back up with breath support. Start with one and work up to three with good form.

- Progress to holding a plank for 5 to 10 seconds with good form. Abdominal engagement is the goal, not forming a perfectly straight line from your head to your toes. Lift your bottom as needed, and stop right away if you feel discomfort, a falling-out sensation, or pain.

- Once you have a stable, controlled plank, put the elements together: roll from standing to a plank and complete one full push-up. Begin with 1 repetition and increase to 3. When you can do 3 repetitions with good form, increase the number of push-ups to 2 and then 3.

- Remember to exhale to coordinate with this movement. Resist the urge to hold your breath, lock your throat, or bear down to make the roll.

DYNAMIC AND STRENGTHENING PILATES EXERCISES

Once you can complete supine, side-lying, prone, and standing exercises with consistency and stability, you can revisit dynamic movements such as Rolling Like a Ball. Olson recommends practicing a controlled half roll while your feet are elevated on a block or a BOSU ball. From there, practice a full roll with a Theraband looped around your feet to increase stability before moving on to the full exercise.

A key Pilates exercise for well-rounded strengthening is the bridge series, including the spinal roll, bridge with a hip hinge, and leg lifting and lowering. Incorporating glute activation into your practice can alleviate back pain and improve functional movement as well as performance in other types of exercise.

RETURNING TO PILATES CLASS

Pilates instructors have to seek out additional education to work specifically with postpartum folks, so you may want to ask your instructor if they've had that training. This is not the same as "I've worked with countless people who have had kids," and the training highlights specific areas of need and modification that you could benefit from. In lieu of a coach or trainer who has had that training, an instructor who moves around the room, offers verbal and physical (with consent) adjustments, proactively shares modifications, and is available for questions before and after class is a high-quality runner-up. One indication that your instructor is up to date in their continuing education is that they no longer use the "belly button to the spine" cue for core activation. Instead, they may say to brace your abdominal muscles, activate your core, or use imagery such as gently wrapping your core (as Olson says, wrap your breakfast burrito, don't squish it!). Access is dictated by geography, so if you have limited options or are taking classes online, use the information here to support your return to practice.

As always, beware the beast of comparison. You may have done Pilates before pregnancy and during pregnancy. You may have expectations for your body and its performance. You may be someone who has never failed to "keep up" before and find that your coordination and speed are reduced, even if bracing your core feels like second nature. The postpartum body is still your body. But it's not the same body that was doing Pilates before. The kind of mentality that says "I'm going to work harder and it's going to be like it was before" is likely to cause injury. Be patient with yourself and the process of regaining your strength, endurance, and coordination. It will come with less risk of injury if you are a patient trainer for yourself and respect where you are every time you come to the mat.

CHAPTER 14

Running

Running is a dynamic cardiovascular activity that relies on single-limb stability and power, including your ankles, knees, hips, pelvis, and spine. It combines elements of aerobic endurance—sustained heart rate and blood pressure changes—as well as strength, coordination, power, and speed with repetitive impact. Many people like running because all you need are your shoes and someplace to run. Your identity, athleticism, and mental health may be tied to running, and it can be difficult to give it up, change it, or adapt from what you are used to. You get to decide what is best for your total well-being. Our job is to inform you of the risk factors. Unfortunately, the evidence is clear that postpartum runners are prone to stress urinary incontinence (SUI) and running-related injury. Are the odds in your favor? If you had SUI before or during pregnancy, high mileage, and/or vaginal/genital birth, your odds of leaking are higher. We don't want to scare you, but rather to offer guidelines for a return to running that will reduce your fear of injury and movement and protect your body as you hit the ground again.

TESTING BASELINE STABILITY: ARE YOU STRONG ENOUGH TO RUN?

Getting back to running without injury or pelvic symptoms relies on your ability to regain pelvic stability, as outlined in chapter 7, "The Lumbopelvic System." Working toward single-leg stability, total body strength, and readiness for impact will allow you to return to running safely. Otherwise, running may cause symptoms you are not experiencing during no/low impact exercises. Work at that stability!

Here is a cheat sheet of exercises:

- 30 repetitions of single-leg heel raise on each leg with good arch control
- 20 repetitions on each leg:
  - Single-leg squat
  - Single-leg bridge with straight leg raise (SLR)
  - Straight leg raise with abduction
  - Dead bug

- PFM 10-second holds, 10 reps in standing and lunge position
- Single-leg dead lift, 10 reps on each leg
- Side plank: forearm to heels 30 to 60 seconds on both sides
- Bird dog: 60 seconds on both sides

RECONDITIONING

Aerobic endurance or cardiovascular fitness is an area you can improve *while* building stability. Experts recommend walking in 5-minute intervals to start, slowly building to at least 30 minutes of regular walking three to five days per week. Your walking should be in the same setting as your runs. We recommend swapping out your shoes from pregnancy or pre-pregnancy to account for changes in foot shape and control and body weight. You should be able to walk without abdominal or pelvic floor symptoms such as leaking, bulging, heaviness, or pain. Secondary symptoms like hip or back pain might also be clues that your musculoskeletal system is not ready to absorb impact or handle repetitive strain. If you feel loose or hypermobile in your pelvic joints, try an SI belt during your walks.

Monitor your heart rate to understand more about your exercise adaptations. Learning you are deconditioned can be a difficult pill to swallow. Many runners who have races and awards under their belts are particularly loath to give in to the reality that their capacity is not what it once was. We know! If you could push through it, you would. You probably have tales of harrowing races you trained for and injuries you've trained through. You have been able to meet your running goals before. Everything is different now. Your heart, lungs, and blood vessels have changed. You are more fatigable. Monitor your resting heart rate, your heart rate max, and your heart rate 10 minutes after exercise. If you wear a fitness tracking device, track your maximum heart rate and see what is happening. How long are you above your 85 percent HR max? Are you able to recover within 10 minutes? Do any pelvic floor or pain symptoms occur when you're hitting that max?

RETURN PLAN

Interval Training

Returning to running should include a plan to run/walk your mileage. Start with intervals of running for 1 minute and walking for 1 to 3 minutes. Your first time, aim for 1 to 2 miles total. Leave time to be able to walk without running if symptoms occur. Find a proportion of walking to running and mileage that is consistently symptom-free; play with the numbers to dial in to where you are right now. Once you find a walk-to-run ratio and mileage that feel okay, give yourself one to two days off from running to recover. Practice that program three to five times consistently before increasing total time, mileage, *or* the run-to-walk ratio. Remember your FITT principles: change either frequency, time, or intensity, not all three at once.

Form

Your form should move your body through space with ease and include hitting the ground with your midfoot or forefoot, never your heels. How quiet can you make your footfalls? How gently can you strike the ground? Leaning forward uses momentum to push yourself through space with good core support (integrate those deep systems!). Leaning backward, in contrast, will increase the pressure on your posterior pelvic floor and can cause fecal urgency (runner's trots, anyone?) or back pain. It will also increase the load on your hip flexors and quads, instead of evenly utilizing all your hip muscles. Leaning back is like hitting the brakes and the gas at the same time. Lean forward at the trunk to improve efficiency and bladder control.

Encourage your lower rib cage to rotate as you swing your arms. An easy cue is to pull your elbow back with every step (same arm as the leg out front). Rib cage rotation loads the obliques and assists with core recoil during your stride. A rotating rib cage can happen without crossing the arms in front of the chest during your stride. Deep inhales that expand the rib cage 360 degrees help with the recoil of the ribs and enhance oxygenation.

Your head should be straight and in line with your body. Imagine someone is pointing a finger at your chin to tuck it down instead of jutting it out. Forward head and chin and a rounded back typically go together. This posture is not ideal, as it reduces the surface area of your heart and lungs, giving them less room to productively oxygenate and move oxygen-rich blood to your working muscles. To compensate for a rounded back, do not arch the mid back and push the ribs forward. Keep the ribs gently stacked over the pelvis. Use the elbow drive, 360-degree inhalation, and gentle chin tuck to correct a poorly held rib cage.

Stroller Use

You may surmise that correcting your rib position and breathing make pushing a stroller ill-advised. Indeed, your form will be affected by pushing a stroller. You can work with this by ensuring the stroller is at the right height for you (if adjustable). Hold the handle with one hand and practice the elbow drive with your free hand. Switch sides during your intervals. Be sure to lean forward to use momentum to drive the stroller. On the side holding the stroller, keep your elbow bent but stiff and lock your wrist in neutral. If you keep the pushing arm stiff, it acts as an effective lever to propel the stroller forward rather than pushing with your upper body and arms. Beware of running with a tucked butt and rounded back, which will increase pelvic floor load and pressure. Test your tolerance on a cesarean birth scar by walking your route with the stroller first, especially if there are hills. Downhill will cause a natural lean back. Uphill will make the stroller heavier and require more power and stiffness from the core.

Intensity or Workload

As you are likely well aware, the workload in running can come from multiple sources. The first is your cadence, or steps per minute (spm). The recommended steps per minute for regular running is 160 to 180. An easy way to train yourself to do this is to take smaller steps. You can set your pace with a playlist of songs at this pace or use a fitness watch to track it for you. Try "Hey Ya!" by Outkast or "Sabotage" by the Beastie Boys for the 160–170 spm range, "Whatta Man" by Salt-N-Pepa and En Vogue or "Runnin' Down a Dream" by Tom Petty and the Heartbreakers for the 170–180 spm range, and "Love Is a Battlefield" by Pat Benatar, "Rock and Roll" by Led Zeppelin, or "Rock Lobster" by the B-52's for songs that will keep you running around 180 spm. Maintaining a consistently high cadence will take more cardiovascular endurance, which is why it's good to do this in interval training to rebuild your capacity with proper form.

Why not slow down the cadence for a lower workload? Fewer steps per minute can cause you to dramatically change your stride. A slow or long stride can cause increased force when you hit the ground, which is more likely to cause negative effects on your body, like pain or leakage. It can also change your form, causing you to strike on your heels, rather than on your midfoot or forefoot, and lean back to slow yourself down. Remember that leaning forward and staying balanced and responsive on your toes will improve your athleticism and reduce pressure on the pelvic floor and bladder, and keeping a good cadence will train you to be a stronger and more capable runner. Increase the time you spend walking if 160–180 spm feels difficult for you.

Treadmill Considerations

Running on a treadmill can alter your form and speed in sneaky ways. Try not to hold on to the machine, or if you must, follow the recommendations for the stroller, changing arms intermittently. It's easy to hit harder on the treadmill than the ground, so focus on quiet footfalls. If you feel like you are leaning back too much, increasing the slope or incline to 3 percent can get your posture correctly dialed in. Ignore the number on the treadmill, and instead increase speed based on your sensation of control each time you run rather than on whatever you ran at last time.

RUNNING WITH STRESS URINARY INCONTINENCE AND PROLAPSE

Despite your best efforts, you may still leak when you run. If you have SUI, try running with a tampon in, which supports the urethra and bladder neck internally to reduce leaks. Other products that assist with bladder support like Poise Impressa bladder supports and the Revive reusable bladder support by Ovala Inc. may be more comfortable but cost slightly more than tampons, and none of these products will stop leaking caused by dehydration, urgency, or constipation. Try to run after your daily BM and do not intake bladder irritants such as caffeinated or carbonated beverages for two hours prior to running. Stay in a steady state of hydration to improve your tolerance to your bladder filling at regular intervals. Should you pee before you run? Maybe, but notice whether it is becoming part of a "just in case" peeing pattern. Try trusting your bladder and working on your breathing and form.

If you have a prolapse, talk to your doctor about a pessary. This will hold the organs up and help you with PFM (pelvic floor muscles) and core reintegration. The feeling of heaviness or bulge from the prolapse may cause you to try to hold tension the entire run. We hope you know by now that this is not recommended or even possible, and it is more likely to increase your symptoms.

Postpartum Humans: NP

PROBLEM

Postpartum incontinence almost stole NP's identity as a runner. She was a first-time parent with a mostly unremarkable vaginal birth, except for her stage 3 perineal tear. She followed the rules laid out to her by her midwife and waited six months before she tried jogging. She didn't leak with a cough/laugh/sneeze, although she did if she took too big a step on walks and hikes. As soon as she ran, she experienced major incontinence. Not being able to run was a devastating loss on top of the "light switch" identity change that came with parenthood.

SOLUTION

NP lost time by avoiding cardio conditioning for six weeks due to initial leakage and fear of injuring her pelvic floor. She was strong and cleared most of the stability training with no problem, but she needed to develop better movement strategies and a tolerance for impact. With support from a pelvic health PT, NP realized her "lack of Kegel" was actually pelvic floor muscle tension. She worked on allowing time and relaxation for regular bowel movements and developing strategies for using physical strength without increasing intra-abdominal pressure (particularly in her work as an ER nurse) or clenching her butt for stability. Her physical therapist helped her focus on running form by developing ankle and glute strategies to propel her body, rather than relying on her back muscles. When she improved her ankle and foot control and her forward lean, she noted immediate differences in her ability to run without leaking.

CHAPTER 15

Kettlebell

Kettlebell is a popular at-home or gym resistance and training activity. Its low cost and easy access make it palatable even during the high demands of the postpartum period. Moving a kettlebell even 15 minutes for three days a week is linked to reduced symptoms of depression and anxiety. The movements in kettlebell are functional and will improve your capacity to lift weights at different angles using almost all your large muscle groups, which trains your ability to lift and carry a weight in space or to lift from the floor (a situation that may be coming up a lot these days!).

For the postpartum practitioner, Coach Damali Fraiser of Lift Off Strength & Wellness suggests building up to a 5-to-10-minute session to start. The frequency of your practice will depend on your workload: a light workout can be done five to seven days per week, moderate three to five days per week, and heavy two to three days per week. The goal is to return to baseline without pain, strain, or symptoms of depletion before you train again.

Traditional kettlebell has a higher proportion of ballistic exercises than other strength training methods do, combining strength with power and speed. We do not recommend starting with these movements, which include cleans, swings, and snatches. Instead, build a consistent foundational practice of moving weight with control before adding speed and power to your lifts. If you need cardiovascular conditioning to prepare for the heart rate changes in the ballistic movements, try biking or walking to build your system back up. Remember to plan the order of operations in your sessions to prioritize your preferred task.

STANCE AND BREATH

To get started, check your static (unmoving) stance. If possible, you should be barefoot to connect with the ground and be able to hold your stance.

Can you hold anatomic neutral in seated? Can you hold anatomic neutral in standing? (Ignore the normal cue to jump out to your standing stance right now; step out wider than normal and feel it out.) These are building your tolerance for creating spine stiffness. Focus on getting your stance postures set, then adding breath.

Kettlebell coach Laura Hmelo Jawad recommends practicing coordinating breath with core and PFM (pelvic floor muscles) activation during both simple movements and movements requiring significant effort. Can you both activate and release tension in your stance? You need to relearn how to match muscle tension to task and breathe throughout the effort (remember, breathing is the signal for reintegration of PFM and core). Coach Damali cautions that while it might seem helpful to wear a brace or corset to add power and tolerance to your lifts, it has the potential to compress your rib cage or core, which would restrict your breath and disconnect you from your core and PFM. A correctly worn SI belt will protect your pelvic joints without interrupting your intra-abdominal pressure (IAP) and breathing in a way that shuts down your system connection.

Next, learn to move with breath control under a load. A farmer's carry while resisting rotation and bending to the side with gentle walking will provide you with information about tension in your body, one-sidedness in the strength of your core or PFM, and your heel-to-toe walking pattern. Consider building consistent duration or time under tension, creating equal effort/strength in the left and right sides, and maintaining the ability to take a deep breath while moving this load. If walking is too much, practice holding asymmetric tension while seated or standing to build your tolerance for strength and time under tension.

To challenge your static stance, practice a slingshot or around the world. Are you able to breathe as you pass the weight from hand to hand? Do you lose arch control and knee position? Can you do the halo more easily (no changing hands)? Compare the two. When you hold the weight down near your legs, is there more or less tolerance in your back, core, and PFM compared to holding the weight high to do the halos? Does your breath change? As these are continuous movements without a clear place to blow before you go or exhale with exertion, they are great exercises to practice your deep inhalation without locking your throat or maintaining too much tension in the chest, ribs, or core.

DEAD LIFTS

Ready for more body movement? Feeling good about your symmetry, breathing, and time under tension? Dead lifts are functional movement patterns (kitchen sink, laundry, changing table) that train your back, hip, and core muscles together. You can start by practicing hip hinging in a chair. PFM-friendly breathing is an inhale during the forward lean (PFM lengthens), exhale on the return (PFM shortens). Progress to standing when your seated dead lifts feel coordinated and pain-free.

Add the kettlebell when you're ready (even to seated). You may not have the range of motion to lift and move the kettlebell to the floor yet, which has to do with muscle control at end range. Bring the floor up to you instead with a bench or yoga block and set the kettlebell on that; then progress to dead lifts from the floor when moving from the block is easy. Watch your stance; remember that you want to turn out without realizing you are doing it. Look down at your feet before you move weight. Not sure what weight to use? Pick one that you can hold easily without upper body symptoms and that starts to challenge your torso and legs at 8 to 12 reps. Working too light might make you create more tension than is necessary. Working too heavy will require more rest days or result in symptoms of heaviness or pain after your workout.

A two-handed dead lift would be the normal starting point, but Coach Damali reminds us that you may have breast/chest/top tissue you did not before. Make sure you have a sports bra or chest compression garment that supports you without restricting your breath. Use a lighter kettlebell in one hand to do a suitcase-carry single-arm dead lift or a single-arm conventional dead lift if that increases the exercise's accessibility. Practice controlled reps on both sides—remember, one-handed exercises will force you to resist side-bending and rotation slightly more.

Can you video your dead lift? This move is foundational to the rest of kettlebell, including cleans, presses, swings, and snatches, and should look straight with equal spine tension. You may not realize you have a funny head and shoulder position (no neck with a forward chin), a rounded upper back (frequently seen in people who are breast/chestfeeding), an overly arched mid to lower back (pregnancy posture and core weakness at play), or a tucked butt instead of a hip hinge (the dreaded mom butt—*cringe*—strikes again). A dead lift involves a straight spine, neutral scapulae, and a lengthening hip/pelvic floor with good leg support. Video yourself and work with and without weight to see if there is a difference before you build more kettlebell exercises.

MIDDLE BODY BUILDS

When you watch your dead-lift video, you may find that all your issues are prominently in one body area. The good news is you can build strength in these areas.

Goblet Squats

To build leg, hip hinge, and butt control, practice goblet squats, which should be two-handed. Make sure you move the elbows away from your breast/top tissue so that you can manage the weight comfortably. Start with a chair hip hinge, holding the weight goblet style. Coordinate an inhale to lean forward, and exhale to sit up straight. Practice moving from the hip hinge to standing from the chair while holding the weight. Slowing down to move from stand to sit will build more gluteal and pelvic muscle control for lengthening. This is the primary issue with a tucked-under bottom. You are trying to shorten the glutes and pelvic floor rather than learning how to lengthen them through a full range of motion to hold your body weight. What are your knees and arches doing? Do you need to add outward pressure to hold them open and stay neutral? Once a goblet squat from the chair feels easy, progress to a regular goblet squat. Remember to breathe.

Bent-Over Rows

Having issues with a rounded back? Can't find the balance between a neutral upper back and a neutral rib cage that doesn't thrust forward? Bent-over rows are a way to build upper back strength for better scapula control. Holding your kettlebell in one hand, get into your dead lift and hold this position. Row a bent elbow back with a neutral wrist. Repeat on both sides. Start double arm rows when you know you can hold neutral dead-lift stance under tension with good breathing and without symptoms. Increase the amount you are "bent over" when you can recover easily after these workouts.

Pallof Press

Having issues with your core dumping forward (an arched lower back and a pronounced roundness to your belly)? Get in your neutral stance, bend your knees, and hold your kettlebell to your chest with both hands. Press the kettlebell away from your body, straightening your elbows as much as your breast/chest/top tissue will allow. This is usually an exhale breath, but you can try the forward lean and blow before you go if that helps your core and PFM set up better under this load. Do this against a wall if you can't hold your rib cage still during the movement.

Biceps Curls

Having a hard time holding shoulder tension or a forward head posture? Have a tendency to lean to one side instead of holding a neutral torso without a bend to the side? Biceps curls are a great way to retrain these issues. Hold the kettlebell in one hand. Practice staying in neutral during the biceps curl without moving your upper body, rib cage, shoulders, or head. Mirrors or video feedback are helpful here. Build symmetry on both sides.

CLEANS

The "cheat clean" is a way to safely lift and develop your ability to move the kettlebell from a low to a racked position. Get into triangle stance (wide anatomical neutral), kettlebell handle pointing straight ahead. Grab the handle with one or both hands—the extra hand can hold the bell instead of the handle during the clean if that is easier—and swing and rack the kettlebell to your shoulder with a straight wrist. Lead with your elbow tucked into your body and punch up. A non-cheat, or regular, clean removes the support of the second arm, either having it rest at your side or holding it straight ahead at chest level.

PRESSES

Clean the kettlebell to the rack position (either cheat or regular). Exhale and press the kettlebell straight overhead. Make sure your wrist is straight from the clean to the press. Do you need to add tension? Did you lose neutral in your posture? Did you sway, bulge, dip, or tilt? Add tension to your core, glutes, and quads. Exhale with exertion or blow before you go to get reflexive core and PFM activation. To build core stability, practice presses in standing, kneeling, and half kneeling to gain control in a variety of positions. You can regress by practicing from seated.

HOW TO PROGRESS AND REGRESS YOUR KETTLEBELL WORKOUTS USING FITT PRINCIPLES

Frequency: days per week or total training time
Intensity:
    Volume: duration of time under tension or reps, sets
    Load: weight and speed of motion
    Position: seated, standing, half kneeling, to kneeling
Time: time under tension or total time with the kettlebell
Type: static with gentle movement versus ballistic/fast movements

RETURNING TO BALLISTIC MOVEMENT: SWINGS AND SNATCHES

Jawad recommends working to develop strength, core stability, and coordination through static movements such as dead lifts, dead bugs, Pallof presses, and planks before attempting to return to ballistic movement. Slowly add load, then increase your speed. Once you are performing your strength-building exercises with excellent form, coordinated breath, and tension that's appropriate to the task, add power. Return to swinging with power swings/dead stop swings and gradually work up to continuous swings.

As you begin to add kettlebell movement, you may find that changes in your body size and shape pose challenges. To make sure your kettlebell won't accidentally bump into a body part that's bigger or a different shape than you're used to, Coach Damali recommends aligning your shoulder with the inside of your knee before starting any kettlebell movement. This alignment allows the kettlebell to move around your body as it is, and it particularly allows room for breast/chest/top tissue.

Other postpartum body shifts can impact your kettlebell practice; for one, your pelvis may now have a forward tilt, which can lead to a tendency to overextend your hips at the top of a swing. Jawad recommends giving your momentum extra attention, stopping your movement when your ears, shoulders, hips, and ankles are aligned to avoid putting extra pressure on your abdominal wall and potentially leading to doming or leaking at the top of a swing. Connect the pubic bone to the ribs, resisting the urge to lean back into the pregnancy posture with a swayback.

Jawad offers the following program to return to kettlebell swings:

Return to Kettlebell Swings

A Three-Phase Program by Laura Jawad, Kettlebell Coach

Note: Remain in each phase until you can perform the prescribed number of reps while breathing and without pain or symptoms. Regress as necessary and feel free to choose exercises from a previous phase to incorporate into your next phase.

MINIMUM EQUIPMENT:
- Lighter set of kettlebells for pushing/pulling exercises
- Heavier kettlebell for dead lifts, squats, and swings
- A long-looped resistance band
- Miniband (optional)
- Resistance band door anchor

PHASE 1

WORKOUT A
3 x 8–10 reps:

1a. Incline push-up
1b. Dead bug
2a. Romanian dead lift (slow tempo)
2b. Half-kneeling overhead press
2c. Half-kneeling Pallof press

WORKOUT B
3 x 8–10 reps:

1a. Incline plank
1b. Straight arm pulldown
2a. Goblet squat
2b. Bent-over row
3. Squat pull-apart

PHASE 2

WORKOUT A
3 x 8–10 reps:

1a. Incline push-up
1b. Band pullover dead bug
2a. Romanian dead lift (quick tempo)
2b. Standing overhead press (one arm)
2c. Split stance Pallof press
3. Push press

WORKOUT B
3 x 8–10 reps:

1a. Push-up plank
1b. Band pulldown, knees up
2a. Offset squat
2b. One-arm row
2c. Front raise
3. Two-arm clean (aka goblet clean, pull catch)

PHASE 3

WORKOUT A
3–5 x 5 reps:

1a. Glute bridge chest press
1b. Box plank (with or without leg extension)
2a. Hip hinge with miniband
2b. Overhead press—two arms
2c. Standing Pallof press
3. Power swing

WORKOUT B
3–5 x 5 reps:

1a. Hardstyle plank
1b. Tall kneeling pulldown
2a. Squat with pulse
2b. Lawn-mower row
2c. Suitcase carry
3. Continuous two-handed kettlebell swing

CHAPTER 16

CrossFit

CrossFit describes itself as "constantly varied functional movement at high intensity," and for many, it's a favorite form of exercise. The competitive environment pushes practitioners to increase their resistance, reps, time, and speed. However, it can also make a postpartum return challenging.

CrossFit trainer and Mom Session coach Ally Leard acknowledges how hard it can be to overcome the "type A athlete brain" and scale back or discontinue certain movements. She recommends taking time to set expectations for what you expect out of fitness after pregnancy: "It's not going to be the same, it's okay for it to be different. It's a journey."

Leard's mantra for the return to CrossFit is "slow is fast." Sticking to the basics—no-intensity movement such as connecting breath and core to lift light weights, standing from a squatting position, or walking up a hill—for as long as it takes to perform them without pain or symptoms will build the foundation you need in order to progress to higher intensity exercises without injury.

Leard offers the following sample workout for the first few months following your return to exercise:

CrossFit Workout for Returning to Exercise

WARM-UP
5 MINUTES MOVING THROUGH:
10 Trunk Twists
10 Slow Air Squats
10 Alternating Side Lunges
1:00 Chest Stretch (each side)

CORE WORK
1. SUPINE MARCH
2 sets of 10

2. WALL SHOULDER TAPS
2 sets of 10

WORKOUT (NOT FOR TIME)
10 MINUTES MOVING THROUGH:
10 Wall Push-Ups
8 Bench Dips
6 Slow Air Squats

Once you've spent time doing this work to reintegrate and reconnect your mind and body, and you aren't experiencing any pain or other symptoms, rebuild strength by adding volume and weight to these movements before returning to higher intensity workouts:

CrossFit Workout with Increased Volume and Weight

WARM-UP

5 MINUTES MOVING THROUGH:

10 Alternating Quad Stretches

10 Alternating Knuckle Draggers

10 Arm Circles Front and Back

1:00 Pigeon Pose (each side)

CORE WORK

1. BANDED BIRD DOG

3 sets of 10

2. BANDED PULL-APART TOE TAPS

3 sets of 10

WORKOUT

5 ROUNDS FOR TIME:

100-meter Dumbbell Farmer's Carry

10 Dumbbell Push Presses

15 Air Squats

After spending time increasing volume and weight without exacerbating any pain or other symptoms, you can add intensity to your program:

CrossFit Workout with Increased Volume, Weight, and Intensity

WARM-UP

5 MINUTES MOVING THROUGH:

30 Alternating Quad Stretches

30 Arm Swings (up and downs/arm hugs)

30 Mountain Climbers (go to a higher surface if you feel pressure or
   coning of your belly)

30 Samsons

STRENGTH

1 DEAD LIFT

5 sets of 5 reps

SUPERSET

with 5 sets of 20 Banded Good Mornings

WORKOUT

ON THE 4:00 FOR 5 ROUNDS:

10 Cal Bike

12 Ring Rows

24 Dead Lifts (light to moderate weight, something you can do in two sets)

ADDRESSING ATHLETE BRAIN

In an exercise environment designed around accruing points, the biggest
challenge to a safe return to CrossFit might be psychological. Gretchen
Gavett, a CrossFit coach who specializes in pregnancy and postpartum
coaching, recommends tracking your progress based on new goals, rather
than PRs you might have achieved prepregnancy. Rather than trying to
max out the number of reps you perform during an AMRAP, for instance,
shift your goal to be performing a certain number of reps with consistent
form and no pain or symptoms.

A positive way to frame this mindset shift is to consider that you're focusing almost exclusively on strengthening and integrating your core. Core-to-extremity movements are foundational to CrossFit, and giving your breath, core, and pelvic floor time to heal will ensure that they're able to power your lifts and jumps in the future.

FIND THE RIGHT SUPPORT SYSTEM

Especially as you return to more intense and complex exercises, working with an informed and understanding coach to set goals and plan modifications is a pretty clear path to a successful and injury-free return to CrossFit. Coaches with pregnancy- and postpartum-specific training are few and far between, so any instructor who takes the time to hear your goals and work with you is a keeper. Friends and classmates with similar experiences are golden, too.

If you find yourself without resources nearby, Ally Leard offers the following steps to return to specific CrossFit high skill or high intensity exercises:

Specific CrossFit High Skill Movements

STEP ONE	STEP TWO	STEP THREE	STEP FOUR	STEP FIVE	HIGH SKILL MOVEMENT
Ring Row	Sit to Stand	Jump and Hang	Jump, Hang, Knees Up	–	Rope Climbs
Ring Row	Ring Dip	Muscle Up Transitions	Kip Swings	Ring Pull-Up	Muscle Ups
Ring Row	Banded Pull-Up	Kip Swings	–	–	Pull-Up/ Chest to Bar
Lying Leg Lift	Hanging Knee Raise	Kip Swing, Knees Up	–	–	Toes to Bar
Push-Up	Handstand Hold	Strict Box HSPU	–	–	Handstand Push-Up

Specific CrossFit High Intensity Movements

STEP ONE	STEP TWO	STEP THREE	HIGH INTENSITY MOVEMENT
Single-leg work (Lunges, Single-Leg Squats, Skater Hops, Plate Jumps)	Walking uphill	Interval running (example: 100-meter jog, 100-meter walk × 5 sets)	Running
Bounding Drills	Plate Hops	Gradually increase box height	Box Jumps
Bounding Drills	Plate Hops	Interval work (example: 10 Single Unders, rest 3 minutes × 5 rounds)	Jump Rope/ Double Unders

EPILOGUE

Dear Postpartum Humans,

We hope that by now you're empowered with knowledge about your body and the changes in its form and function as a result of pregnancy. You know how and when to access healthcare for pain or symptoms, including emergencies. You've learned exercises to heal and restore function to body systems and have a greater understanding of how your body works together as an integrated whole. You have tools to do cost-benefit analyses for decisions that affect your quality of life and can make choices that have the best outcome for your mental and physical health. You can set function and fitness goals that take into consideration your body just as it is this minute.

We know that this book can't repair broken systems like racial inequity, lack of childcare and parental leave, for-profit insurance plans, and a paucity of research about postpartum bodies. For now, we want to help you work within these crummy systems, but we're hopeful that by breaking down the walls of secrecy around the postpartum period and democratizing access to this information, authentic conversations about the impact pregnancy has on bodies and minds can finally occur. This might even lead to real change.

We can't predict the future, but we can leave you with one final reminder: take a deep breath, let your belly and pelvic floor relax, and take a nice sip of water. No matter how you end this book, remember that you are enough. You have always been enough. Your function postpartum does not determine your worth as a person or as a parent. We want to help you get back to doing what you want to do and living how you want to live. If we didn't cover that here, we hope you find guidance in your usual support systems or within yourself to get there.

ACKNOWLEDGMENTS

The process of this book coming into being has been one of conception, growth, evolution, support, midwifery, and birth. We are so thankful to the island of North Haven, Maine, for being the birthplace of our friendship and therefore of this book. Some things just seem to happen in the right place at the right time, and North Haven has been the right place for many things!

Thank you to Hannah, Anna, and Nina, the NaNaNas, our group of publishing know-hows who fostered the idea of this book into the perfect creation you now hold in your hands: Anna Worrall for being our person in the know, telling Courtney "This is the one!" and delivering our book baby into the publishing world; Nina Shield for saying YES, this needs to happen, and giving us hilarious play-by-play feedback as she navigated her own immediate postpartum recovery; and Hannah Steigmeyer for gently shaping this book to be digestible and important material for you.

We interviewed so many people for this book. Thank you to the postpartum humans who shared their stories with us. Thank you to the professionals who shared their time and expertise: Dr. Damali Campbell, Dr. Jay Naliboff, Dr. Lauren Naliboff, Dr. Julia McDonald, Julie Wiebe, PT, Amanda Olson, DPT, PRPC, Dustienne Miller, PT, MS, WCS, CYT, Paula Norcott, IBCLC, Suzie Zimmerman, CNM, Molly McBride, Regina Tricamo, LCSW, Elizabeth Theriault, Lindsey Piper, Coach Damali Fraiser, Laura Jawad, Courtney Wyckoff, Brianna

Bedigian, Ally Leard, and Gretchen Gavett. Thank you to Trystan Reese for expounding upon your trans parent experience.

Thank you to our children, Pen and Sam, for allowing us to tell any part of their birth stories.

From Ruth:

I would like to thank my spouse, Adam, for his sperm contribution, not passing out during our kid's birth, summers spent on North Haven, hot dinners during long weeks, strong encouragement, never once making me feel like my postpartum body needed to be gotten over, scoffing at the "hot dog up the hallway" myth, and in general being an original, wonderful, expansive partner who encourages me to be my most authentic self in every iteration. Thank you to Tracy for being my sounding board: our calls are still a highlight of my day. Sharon gets all the kudos for time-outs involving hot tubs, snowshoeing, bowling, time on the lake, walks, and generally getting away from the computer to get my head straight. Thank you to my sister Hannah for believing in me, always being a force for good, and raising some exceptional humans. Thank you to my aunties for sending me messages, keeping it real, and clapping from afar! Dr. Melissa Streeter, you remain my work mentor and biggest supporter! Thank you for elevating pelvic health in our healthcare system and supporting people to get care for things other docs kept saying were "normal." Thank you to Krystyna Holland and Laurel Proulx for reading the book proposal and not thinking I was insane! Cora Huitt, you told me when I was a twenty-three-year-old PT student that I was made to do pelvic health work. I didn't believe you, but you planted a seed that took time to grow! Thank you to my pelvic health coworkers for your support in our collective work and its evolution: Catherine Jaquith, Charlotte Leary, Hallie Sikes, Sarah Geis, Jen Wolfe, Rebecca Brewster-Taylor, and Morgan Cooper. Thank you to Yonca Berk-Giray for your constant "lips to hips" feedback on our shared SLP and pelvic health patients. Courtney, you have been an exceptional progenitor of *Your Postpartum Body*. Thanks for trusting me to be a good steward in improving postpartum life for all humans and meeting deadlines (even if by the skin of my teeth). Your grace under pressure is truly admirable. Thank you from the bottom of my heart to every patient who has ever entrusted their care and their stories to my hands and my heart. This book is for you, most of all.

From Courtney:

Infinite gratitude is due to Penrose and Bill, without whom I wouldn't be a postpartum human, and who make me want to make the world a better place. My parents, Dr. Jay and Jane Naliboff, and sisters, Dr. Lauren and Dana Naliboff, offered invaluable expertise and suggestions, both medical and authorly, and let me talk and text through the research and writing process. To Fiona Robins and Claire Donnelly, Bait Bags for life, thank you for letting me process my birth experience through song and find a first home for the realization that "nobody told me!" To Mitch Zuckoff and Mara Altman, thank you for giving me the tools and permission to be a writer. I know we thanked Anna Worrall, our amazing agent at the Gernert Company, above, but I needed to shout her out here, too—if she hadn't graciously read (and rejected) another book proposal as a favor to a fellow North Havener, we wouldn't be here today. And of course I'm so grateful to Ruth, whose expertise I benefited from long before this book was a twinkle in its parents' eyes. If you hadn't agreed to be my coauthor, *Your Postpartum Body* might have stayed a Google Doc list of my bodily dysfunctions forever.

We have benefited from an expansive village and community to bring this book to your hands. The world is full of "invisible" work that keeps us going, keeps us focused, and keeps us motivated. No work is done in isolation. We are thankful to everyone working in the birthing and postpartum industries, whether through direct care, advocacy, or research. Your work may feel forgotten, but it is not. Keep fighting the good fight. We need you.

NOTES

Chapter 1. Caring for the Postpartum Body and Mind

6. **Your feet flatten:** Neil A. Segal et al., "Pregnancy Leads to Lasting Changes in Foot Structure," *American Journal of Physical Medicine & Rehabilitation* 92, no. 3 (2013): 232–40, https://doi.org/10.1097/phm.0b013e31827443a9.

10. **Mental health issues occur:** Maternal Mental Health Leadership Alliance, "Fact Sheet: Maternal Mental Health (MMH)," https://www.mmhla.org/fact-sheets.

13. **improved cognitive function, attention, memory, and mood:** Natalie A. Masento et al., "Effects of Hydration Status on Cognitive Performance and Mood," *British Journal of Nutrition* 111, no. 10 (2014): 1841–52, https://doi.org/10.1017/S000711 4513004455.

13. **How much water:** Contributor(s): Institute of Medicine; Food and Nutrition Board; Panel on Dietary Reference Intakes for Electrolytes and Water; Standing Committee on the Scientific Evaluation of Dietary Reference Intakes, *Dietary Reference Intakes for Water, Potassium, Sodium, Chloride, and Sulfate* (Washington, DC: National Academies Press, 2005), https://doi.org/10.17226/10925.

15. **overall hydration and muscle recovery:** Rick L. Sharp, "Role of Whole Foods in Promoting Hydration After Exercise in Humans," *Journal of the American College of Nutrition* 26, supp. 5 (2007), https://doi.org/10.1080/07315724.2007.10719664.

16. **8,000 to 10,000 calories per day:** OlympicTalk, "How Many Calories Michael Phelps Consumed as a Swimmer," OlympicTalk, NBC Sports, May 5, 2020, https://olympics.nbcsports.com/2020/05/05/michael-phelps-calories-swimming/#:~:text=Michael%20Phelps%20liked%20to%20say,ten%20thousand%20calories%20per%20day.%E2%80%9D.

17. **fiber per day:** Holly R. Hull et al., "The Effect of High Dietary Fiber Intake on Gestational Weight Gain, Fat Accrual, and Postpartum Weight Retention: A Randomized Clinical Trial," *BMC Pregnancy and Childbirth* 20, no. 1 (2020): article 319, https://doi.org/10.1186/s12884-020-03016-5.

17. **Recommended amounts of protein:** Michelle A. Kominiarek and Priya Rajan,

"Nutrition Recommendations in Pregnancy and Lactation," *Medical Clinics of North America* 100, no. 6 (2016): 1199–215, https://doi.org/10.1016/j.mcna.2016 .06.004.

17. **grams of protein for every kilogram of body weight:** Betina Rasmussen et al., "Protein Requirements of Healthy Lactating Women Are Higher Than the Current Recommendations," *Current Developments in Nutrition* 4, supp. 2 (2020): 653, https:// doi.org/10.1093/cdn/nzaa049_046.

21. **Postpartum thyroiditis, a condition:** Maria M. Fariduddin and Gurdeep Singh, "Thyroiditis—StatPearls," NCBI Bookshelf, National Library of Medicine, https:// www.ncbi.nlm.nih.gov/books/NBK555975.

23. **milk comes in:** "Session 2: The Physiological Basis of Breastfeeding," from *Infant and Young Child Feeding: Model Chapter for Textbooks for Medical Students and Allied Health Professionals* (Geneva: World Health Organization, 2009), https:// www.ncbi.nlm.nih.gov/books/NBK148970.

26. **milk removal sessions:** Jacqueline C. Kent, Danielle K. Prime, and Catherine P. Garbin, "Principles for Maintaining or Increasing Breast Milk Production," *Journal of Obstetric, Gynecologic & Neonatal Nursing* 41, no. 1 (2012): 114–21, https://doi .org/10.1111/j.1552-6909.2011.01313.x.

29. **taking lecithin to prevent recurring blockages:** "Lecithin—Drugs and Lactation Database (LactMed)," NCBI Bookshelf, National Library of Medicine, https:// www.ncbi.nlm.nih.gov/books/NBK501772.

29. **Breast/Chest Lymph Massage:** Nutchanat Munsittikul et al., "Integrated Breast Massage Versus Traditional Breast Massage for Treatment of Plugged Milk Duct in Lactating Women: A Randomized Controlled Trial," *International Breastfeeding Journal* 17, no. 43 (2022): article 43, https://doi.org/10.1186/s13006-022 -00485-6.

35. **traumatic birth story:** Julián Rodríguez-Almagro et al., "Women's Perceptions of Living a Traumatic Childbirth Experience and Factors Related to a Birth Experience," *International Journal of Environmental Research and Public Health* 16, no. 9 (2019): 1654, https://doi.org/10.3390/ijerph16091654.

36. **perinatal post-traumatic stress disorder:** Burcu Kömürcü Akik and Ayşegül Durak Batıgün, "Perinatal Post Traumatic Stress Disorder Questionnaire-II (PPQ-II): Adaptation, Validity, and Reliability Study," *Dusunen Adam: The Journal of Psychiatry and Neurological Sciences* 33, no. 4 (2020): 340–50, https://doi.org/10.14744/dajpns .2020.00102.

36. **perinatal or postpartum PTSD:** Cheryl Tatano Beck, Sue Watson, and Robert K. Gable, "Traumatic Childbirth and Its Aftermath: Is There Anything Positive?," *Journal of Perinatal Education* 27, no. 3 (2018): 175–84, https://doi.org/10.1891/1058 -1243.27.3.175.

36. ***Mothering from Your Center*:** Tami Lynn Kent, *Mothering from Your Center: Tap-*

ping Your Body's Natural Energy for Pregnancy, Birth, and Parenting (New York: Atria Paperback, 2013).

36. **David Grand's *Brainspotting*:** David Grand, *Brainspotting: The Revolutionary New Therapy for Rapid and Effective Change* (Boulder, CO: Sounds True, 2013).

38. **herbal teas if lactating:** Karen Miles, "Herbs and Herbal Teas to Avoid While Breastfeeding," BabyCenter, August 31, 2022, https://www.babycenter.com/baby /breastfeeding/breast-milk-interactions-chart_8788.

38. **Kimberly Ann Johnson:** Kimberly Ann Johnson, *The Fourth Trimester: A Postpartum Guide to Healing Your Body, Balancing Your Emotions, and Restoring Your Vitality* (Boulder, CO: Shambhala Publications, 2017).

39. ***All The Rage*:** Darcy Lockman, *All the Rage: Mothers, Fathers, and the Myth of Equal Partnership* (New York: Harper Perennial, 2020).

39. **mental and physical health:** Rebekah Edie et al., "Barriers to Exercise in Postpartum Women: A Mixed-Methods Systematic Review," *Journal of Women's Health: Physical Therapy* 45, no. 2 (2021): 83–92, https://doi.org/10.1097/JWH.000000 0000000201.

Chapter 2. Six Weeks

47. **Emily and Amelia Nagoski:** Emily Nagoski and Amelia Nagoski, "Do You Judge Your Own Body? Here's How to View It with Love, Not Shame," ideas.ted.com, March 28, 2019, https://ideas.ted.com/if-youre-unhappy-with-your-body-just -repeat-after-us-you-are-the-new-hotness.

48. **lift your head off the floor:** Nadia Keshwani and Linda McLean, "Ultrasound Imaging in Postpartum Women with Diastasis Recti: Intrarater Between-Session Reliability," *Journal of Orthopaedic & Sports Physical Therapy* 45, no. 9 (2015): 713–18, https://doi.org/10.2519/jospt.2015.5879.

52. **likelihood of tearing or an episiotomy:** Mattea Romano et al., "Postpartum Period: Three Distinct but Continuous Phases," *Journal of Prenatal Medicine* 4, no. 2 (2010): 22–25, https://www.ncbi.nlm.nih.gov/pmc/articles/PMC3279173.

Chapter 3. Postpartum Healthcare

58. **crisis in maternal mortality and morbidity:** Munira Z. Gunja, Evan D. Gumas, and Reginald D. Williams II, "The U.S. Maternal Mortality Crisis Continues to Worsen: An International Comparison," *To the Point* (blog), Commonwealth Fund, December 1, 2022, https://doi.org/10.26099/8vem-fc65.

58. **CDC data reveals:** Donna L. Hoyert, "Maternal Mortality Rates in the United States, 2020," NCHS Health E-Stats, Centers for Disease Control and Prevention, February 23, 2022, https://doi.org/10.15620/cdc:113967, https://www.cdc.gov /nchs/data/hestat/maternal-mortality/2020/maternal-mortality-rates-2020.htm.

58. **focus on the baby rather than on the pregnant person:** "The Surgeon General's

Call to Action to Improve Maternal Health: Executive Summary," https://www.hhs
.gov/sites/default/files/executive-summary-to-improve-maternal-health.pdf.

59. **denial, delay, and dismissal:** Lisa Gittens-Williams and Damali Campbell-Oparaji,
"2/1/22 Medicine Grand Rounds—Dr. Gittens-Williams and Dr. Campbell-Oparaji,"
YouTube, February 4, 2022, https://www.youtube.com/watch?v=ajLUQS_W6U4.

59. **CDC's Hear Her campaign:** "HEAR HER Campaign," Centers for Disease Control
and Prevention, November 17, 2022, https://www.cdc.gov/hearher/index.html.

60. **5 percent of postpartum psychosis cases:** "Postpartum Psychosis," Postpartum
Support International (PSI), February 8, 2023, https://www.postpartum.net/learn
-more/postpartum-psychosis.

60. **if you had gestational diabetes:** Alexis Shub et al., "The Effect of Breastfeeding on
Postpartum Glucose Tolerance and Lipid Profiles in Women with Gestational Diabetes Mellitus," *International Breastfeeding Journal* 14 (2019): article 46, https://
doi.org/10.1186/s13006-019-0238-5.

60. **increased thirst, urination, exhaustion:** "Gestational Diabetes," Mayo Clinic,
April 9, 2022, https://www.mayoclinic.org/diseases-conditions/gestational-diabetes
/symptoms-causes/syc-20355339.

60. **Clotting disorders:** Julie S. Moldenhauer, "Blood Clots After Delivery (Postpartum
Blood Clots)," Merck Manual Consumer Version, last modified September 2022,
https://www.merckmanuals.com/home/women-s-health-issues/postpartum-care
/blood-clots-after-delivery#:~:text=(Postpartum%20Blood%20Clots)&text=Blood
%20clots%20may%20also%20develop,red%2C%20swollen%2C%20and%20
painful.

60. **Sepsis:** "Pregnancy & Childbirth," Sepsis Alliance, March 3, 2023, https://www
.sepsis.org/sepsisand/pregnancy-childbirth.

61. **Peripartum cardiomyopathy:** Denise Hilfiker-Kleiner and Karen Sliwa, "Patho-
physiology and Epidemiology of Peripartum Cardiomyopathy," *Nature Reviews:
Cardiology* 11, no. 6 (2014): 364–70, https://doi.org/10.1038/nrcardio.2014.37.

61. **Myocardial infarction (MI):** H. Lameijer et al., "Pregnancy-Related Myocardial
Infarction." *Netherlands Heart Journal* 25, no. 6 (2017): 365–69, https://doi.org/10
.1007/s12471-017-0989-9.

61. **Stroke:** "Pregnancy-Related Stroke," NewYork-Presbyterian, https://www.nyp.org
/neuro/stroke/pregnancy-related-stroke#:~:text=Pregnancy%20and%20Post
partum%20Stroke%20Symptoms&text=Sudden%20numbness%20or%20weak
ness%20in,that%20occurs%20out%20of%20nowhere.

61. **Breast cancer:** Joe Rojas-Burke, "Study Confirms the Unique Danger of Postpartum Breast Cancers," OHSU News, October 14, 2022, https://news.ohsu.edu/2022
/10/14/study-confirms-the-unique-danger-of-postpartum-breast-cancers
#:~:text=Breast%20cancers%20that%20emerge%20within,factor%20for%20
breast%20cancer%20progression.

61. **new *painless* mass:** "Pregnancy and Breast Cancer—Everything You Need to Know," Breast Care Center Miami, January 14, 2020, https://www.toplinemd.com /breast-care-center-of-miami/blog/pregnancy-and-breast-cancer-everything-you -need-to-know.

62. **what services you need:** Sarah Verbiest et al., "Elevating Mothers' Voices: Recommendations for Improved Patient-Centered Postpartum," *Journal of Behavioral Medicine* 41, no. 5 (2018): 577–90, https://doi.org/10.1007/s10865-018 -9961-4.

63. **Physical therapy (PT):** Claire J. C. Critchley, "Physical Therapy Is an Important Component of Postpartum Care in the Fourth Trimester," *Physical Therapy* 102, no. 5 (2022), https://doi.org/10.1093/ptj/pzac021.

64. **Occupational therapy . . . Postpartum depression:** Skye P. Barbic et al., "Scoping Review of the Role of Occupational Therapy in the Treatment of Women with Postpartum Depression," *Annals of International Occupational Therapy* 4, no. 4 (2021): e249–e259, https://doi.org/10.3928/24761222-20210921-02.

64. **Occupational therapy . . . Breastfeeding support:** Lauren Sponseller, Fern Silverman, and Pamela Roberts, "Exploring the Role of Occupational Therapy with Mothers Who Breastfeed," *American Journal of Occupational Therapy* 75, no. 5 (2021): 7505205110, https://doi.org/10.5014/ajot.2021.041269.

64. **Chiropractic:** Carol Ann Weis et al., "Best-Practice Recommendations for Chiropractic Care for Pregnant and Postpartum Patients: Results of a Consensus Process," *Journal of Manipulative & Physiological Therapeutics* 45, no. 7 (2022): 469–89, https://doi.org/10.1016/j.jmpt.2021.03.002.

65. **Osteopathy:** Victoria Hastings et al., "Efficacy of Osteopathic Manipulative Treatment for Management of Postpartum Pain," *Journal of Osteopathic Medicine* 116, no. 8 (2016): 502–9, https://doi.org/10.7556/jaoa.2016.103.

65. **Osteopathy . . . Back pain:** Florian Schwerla et al., "Osteopathic Manipulative Therapy in Women with Postpartum Low Back Pain and Disability: A Pragmatic Randomized Controlled Trial," *Journal of Osteopathic Medicine* 115, no. 7 (2015): 416–25, https://doi.org/10.7556/jaoa.2015.087.

65. **Acupuncture . . . Pain:** Bing-Shu He, Yang Li, and Tong Gui, "Preliminary Clinical Evaluation of Acupuncture Therapy in Patients with Postpartum Sciatica," *Journal of Midwifery & Women's Health* 63, no. 2 (2018): 214–20, https://doi.org/10.1111 /jmwh.12681.

65. **Acupuncture . . . Postpartum depression:** Shanshan Li et al., "Effectiveness of Acupuncture in Postpartum Depression: A Systematic Review and Meta-Analysis," *Acupuncture in Medicine* 36, no. 5 (2018): 295–301, https://doi.org/10.1136/acup med-2017-011530.

65. **Massage therapy . . . Depression:** Masumi Imura, Hanako Misao, and Hiroshi Ushijima, "The Psychological Effects of Aromatherapy-Massage in Healthy Post-

partum Mothers," *Journal of Midwifery & Women's Health* 51, no. 2 (2006): e21–e27, https://doi.org/10.1016/j.jmwh.2005.08.009.

67. **multiple available providers:** Laura A. Siminoff, "Incorporating Patient and Family Preferences into Evidence-Based Medicine," *BMC Medical Informatics and Decision Making* 13 (2013): article S6, https://doi.org/10.1186/1472-6947-13-s3-s6.

68. **shares life experiences with you:** Kathryn Wouk et al., "A Systematic Review of Patient-, Provider-, and Health System–Level Predictors of Postpartum Health Care Use by People of Color and Low-Income and/or Uninsured Populations in the United States," *Journal of Women's Health* 30, no. 8 (2021): 1127–59, https://doi.org/10.1089/jwh.2020.8738.

68. **positive patient-provider relationship:** Matthew Asare et al., "The Patient–Provider Relationship: Predictors of Black/African American Cancer Patients' Perceived Quality of Care and Health Outcomes," *Health Communication* 35, no. 10 (2020): 1289–94, https://doi.org/10.1080/10410236.2019.1625006.

73. **Herman & Wallace Pelvic Rehabilitation Institute:** "Find a Pelvic Rehabilitation Practitioner," Pelvic Rehab, https://pelvicrehab.com.

73. **APTA-Pelvic Health Section:** "PT Locator: Find a Physical Therapist Near You," APTA Pelvic Health, https://aptapelvichealth.org/ptlocator.

74. **Pregnancy & Postpartum Certified Exercise Specialist:** "Pregnancy and Postpartum Corrective Exercise Specialist Certification Experts," Core Exercise Solutions, https://www.coreexercisesolutions.com/pces-directory.

74. **Julie Wiebe, PT:** "Find-a-Pro," Julie Wiebe PT, July 24, 2019, https://www.juliewiebept.com/professionals-map.

74. **Tracy Sher, PT:** "Pelvic Guru Directory Search," Pelvic Guru, https://pelvicguru.com/directory.

74. **Women of Color Pelvic Floor PT Directory:** "WOC PFPT Directory," Vagina Rehab Doctor, https://www.vaginarehabdoctor.com/woc-pfpt-directory.

74. **Lynn Schulte, PT:** Directory, Institute for Birth Healing, https://directory.instituteforbirthhealing.com.

74. **2020 findings by the CDC:** "Infographic: Identifying Maternal Depression," Centers for Disease Control and Prevention, May 2, 2022, https://www.cdc.gov/reproductivehealth/vital-signs/identifying-maternal-depression/index.html.

77. **medication-assisted recovery model—for example, MaineMOM:** "MaineMOM," Office of MaineCare Services, State of Maine Department of Health and Human Services, https://www.maine.gov/dhhs/oms/about-us/projects-initiatives/mainemom.

Chapter 4. Breathing

87. **Respiration is both:** Antonella LoMauro and Andrea Aliverti, "Respiratory Physiology of Pregnancy," *Breathe* 11, no. 4 (2015): 297–301, https://doi.org/10.1183/20734735.008615.

88. **strengthening and retraining the muscles:** Amrita L. Tomar and Manisha A. Rathi, "Effect of Breathing Exercises on Lung Functions in Postpartum Mothers with Normal Vaginal Delivery," *Indian Journal of Physiotherapy and Occupational Therapy* 8, no. 4 (2014): 248, https://www.researchgate.net/publication/284423733 _Effect_of_Breathing_Exercises_on_Lung_Functions_in_Postpartum_Mothers _with_Normal_Vaginal_Delivery.

88. **the respiratory system is affected:** Antonella LoMauro et al., "Adaptation of Lung, Chest Wall, and Respiratory Muscles During Pregnancy: Preparing for Birth," *Journal of Applied Physiology* 127, no. 6 (2019): 1640–50, https://doi.org/10.1152 /japplphysiol.00035.2019.

94. **reduced symptoms of anxiety, depression, and post-traumatic stress disorder (PTSD):** Xiao Ma et al., "The Effect of Diaphragmatic Breathing on Attention, Negative Affect and Stress in Healthy Adults," *Frontiers in Psychology* 8 (2017): 874, https://doi.org/10.3389/fpsyg.2017.00874.

Chapter 5. Posture

112. **one leg longer than the other:** Gary A. Knutson, "Anatomic and Functional Leg-Length Inequality: A Review and Recommendation for Clinical Decision-Making. Part I, Anatomic Leg-Length Inequality: Prevalence, Magnitude, Effects and Clinical Significance," *Chiropractic & Osteopathy* 13 (2005): article 11, https://doi.org /10.1186/1746-1340-13-11.

118. **Neutral Lying Exercises . . . Decompression:** Katy Bowman, *Diastasis Recti: The Whole-Body Solution to Abdominal Weakness and Separation* (Washington: Propriometrics Press, 2016).

Chapter 6. The Pelvic Floor

126. **Dr. Arnold Kegel, a gynecologist:** Yi-Chen Huang and Ke-Vin Chang, "Kegel Exercises—StatPearls," NCBI Bookshelf, National Library of Medicine, https:// pubmed.ncbi.nlm.nih.gov/32310358.

126. **muscle reeducation to reduce leaking:** Arnold H. Kegel, "Progressive Resistance Exercise in the Functional Restoration of the Perineal Muscles," *American Journal of Obstetrics and Gynecology* 56, no. 2 (1948): 238–48, https://doi.org/10.1016 /0002-9378(48)90266-X.

127. **Morris, a movement instructor:** "Maternity and Post-Operative Exercises in Diagrams and Words," *Journal of the American Medical Association* 108, no. 25 (1937): 2161, https://doi.org/10.1001/jama.1937.02780250075028.

127. **research suggests that only 30 percent:** Míriam Raquel Diniz Zanetti et al., "Impact of Supervised Physiotherapeutic Pelvic Floor Exercises for Treating Female Stress Urinary Incontinence," *São Paulo Medical Journal* 125, no. 5 (2007): 265–69, https://doi.org/10.1590/s1516-31802007000500003.

127. **As Morris and Randell describe it:** Margaret Morris and Minnie Randell, *Maternity and Post-operative Exercises in Diagrams and Words* (New York: Oxford University Press, 1936).

134. **increased sexual distress:** Gracielle C. Schwenck et al., "A Comparison of the Sexual Well-Being of New Parents with Community Couples," *Journal of Sexual Medicine* 17, no. 11 (2020): 2156–67, https://doi.org/10.1016/j.jsxm.2020.08.011.

136. **expect a partner:** Angela Towne, "Clitoral Stimulation During Penile-Vaginal Intercourse: A Phenomenological Study Exploring Sexual Experiences in Support of Female Orgasm," *Canadian Journal of Human Sexuality* 28, no. 1 (2019): 68–80, https://doi.org/10.3138/cjhs.2018-0022.

151. **can produce *vaginal wind*:** Helena Frawley et al., "An International Continence Society (ICS) Report on the Terminology for Pelvic Floor Muscle Assessment," *Neurourology and Urodynamics* 40, no. 5 (2021): 1217–60, https://doi.org/10.1002/nau.24658.

155. **Introduction to the Pelvic Brace:** Leslie M. Parker, *The Art of Control: A Woman's Guide to Bladder Care* (CreateSpace Independent Publishing Platform, 2015).

Chapter 7. The Lumbopelvic System

164. **pelvic girdle pain (PGP):** Susan C. Clinton et al., "Pelvic Girdle Pain in the Antepartum Population: Physical Therapy Clinical Practice Guidelines Linked to the International Classification of Functioning, Disability, and Health from the Section on Women's Health and the Orthopaedic Section of the American Physical Therapy Association," *Journal of Women's Health: Physical Therapy* 41, no. 2 (2017): 102–25, https://doi.org/10.1097/JWH.0000000000000081.

164. **your mental and physical well-being:** Małgorzata Starzec-Proserpio et al., "Association Among Pelvic Girdle Pain, Diastasis Recti Abdominis, Pubic Symphysis Width, and Pain Catastrophizing: A Matched Case–Control Study," *Physical Therapy* 102, no. 4 (2022), https://doi.org/10.1093/ptj/pzab311.

Chapter 8. The Core

174. **sciatica can be caused by positioning:** Sarmistha Roy et al., "Intraoperative Positioning During Cesarean as a Cause of Sciatic Neuropathy," *Obstetrics & Gynecology* 99, no. 4 (2002): 652–53, https://doi.org/10.1016/s0029-7844(01)01700-8.

189. **thinner cross section:** Mako Fukano et al., "Recovery of Abdominal Muscle Thickness and Contractile Function in Women After Childbirth," *International Journal of Environmental Research and Public Health* 18, no. 4 (2021): 2130, https://doi.org/10.3390/ijerph18042130.

189. **called a diastasis recti:** M. Cavalli et al., "Prevalence and Risk Factors for Diastasis Recti Abdominis: A Review and Proposal of a New Anatomical Variation," *Hernia* 25, no. 4 (2021), https://doi.org/10.1007/s10029-021-02468-8; Nicole F. Hills,

Ryan B. Graham, and Linda McLean, "Comparison of Trunk Muscle Function Between Women With and Without Diastasis Recti Abdominis at 1 Year Postpartum," *Physical Therapy* 98, no. 10 (2018): 891–901, https://doi.org/10.1093/ptj/pzy083; Małgorzata Starzec-Proserpio et al., "Association Among Pelvic Girdle Pain, Diastasis Recti Abdominis, Pubic Symphysis Width, and Pain Catastrophizing: A Matched Case–Control Study," *Physical Therapy* 102, no. 4 (2022), https://doi.org/10.1093/ptj/pzab311.

207. **Side Planks . . . Forearm to knee plank:** Deydre S. Teyhen et al., "Changes in Deep Abdominal Muscle Thickness During Common Trunk-Strengthening Exercises Using Ultrasound Imaging," *Journal of Orthopaedic & Sports Physical Therapy* 38, no. 10 (2008): 596–605, https://doi.org/10.2519/jospt.2008.2897.

Chapter 9. The Feet

211. **tendons in your foot, causing pronation:** Marc J. Heronemus et al., "The Association of Parity with Greater Dynamic Pronation of the Feet," *PM&R* 13, no. 2 (2020): 144–52, https://doi.org/10.1002/pmrj.12381.

211. **increased rotation at the knee:** Stacey R. Chu et al., "Pregnancy Results in Lasting Changes in Knee Joint Laxity," *PM&R* 11, no. 2 (2019): 117–24, https://doi.org/10.1016/j.pmrj.2018.06.012.

211. **poor sense of proprioception:** Liliam F. Oliveira et al., "Postural Sway Changes During Pregnancy: A Descriptive Study Using Stabilometry," *European Journal of Obstetrics & Gynecology and Reproductive Biology* 147, no. 1 (2009): 25–28, https://doi.org/10.1016/j.ejogrb.2009.06.027.

Chapter 10. Putting It All Together

231. **Stretching before an activity:** Stephen B. Thacker et al.,"The Impact of Stretching on Sports Injury Risk: A Systematic Review of the Literature," *Medicine & Science in Sports & Exercise* 36, no. 3 (2004): 371–78, https://doi.org/10.1249/01.mss.0000117134.83018.f7.

241. **Impact Readiness Checklist:** Grainne Donnelly, Emma Brockwell, and Tom Goom, "Return to Running Postnatal—Guideline for Medical, Health and Fitness Professionals Managing This Population," *Physiotherapy* 107 (2020): e188–e189, https://doi.org/10.1016/j.physio.2020.03.276.

242. **Strength Readiness Checklist:** Shefali Mathur Christopher et al., "Rehabilitation of the Postpartum Runner: A 4-Phase Approach," *Journal of Women's Health: Physical Therapy* 46, no. 2 (2022): 73–86, https://doi.org/10.1097/jwh.0000000000000230.

243. **You Shall Not Pass: Contraindications:** Jack T. Andrish, "Screening for Sports Participation," Merck Manual Professional Version, September 2022, https://www.merckmanuals.com/professional/injuries-poisoning/sports-injury/screening-for-sports-participation.

243. **Precautions for Return to Sports:** Meredith L. Birsner and Cynthia Gyamfi-Bannerman, "Physical Activity and Exercise During Pregnancy and the Postpartum Period," ACOG Committee Opinion No. 804, April 2020, https://www.acog.org/clinical/clinical-guidance/committee-opinion/articles/2020/04/physical-activity-and-exercise-during-pregnancy-and-the-postpartum-period.

243. **Hypertension: blood pressure above 200 mm Hg:** James E. Sharman, Andre La Gerche, and Jeff S. Coombes, "Exercise and Cardiovascular Risk in Patients with Hypertension," *American Journal of Hypertension* 28, no. 2 (2015): 147–58, https://doi.org/10.1093/ajh/hpu191.

243. **RED-S: relative energy deficiency:** Margo Mountjoy et al., "The IOC Consensus Statement: Beyond the Female Athlete Triad—Relative Energy Deficiency in Sport (RED-S)," *British Journal of Sports Medicine* 48, no. 7 (2014): 491–97, https://doi.org/10.1136/bjsports-2014-093502; Margo Mountjoy et al., "Authors' 2015 Additions to the IOC Consensus Statement: Relative Energy Deficiency in Sport (RED-S)," *British Journal of Sports Medicine* 49, no. 7 (2015): 417–20, https://doi.org/10.1136/bjsports-2014-094371.

243. **female athlete triad syndrome:** Mountjoy et al., "Authors' 2015 Additions to the IOC Consensus Statement: Relative Energy Deficiency in Sport (Red-S)."

Chapter 12. Yoga

257. **Ashtanga yoga (*ashtanga* literally means eight limbs):** Mara Carrico, "Get to Know the 8 Limbs of Yoga," *Yoga Journal,* March 23, 2021, https://www.yogajournal.com/yoga-101/philosophy/8-limbs-of-yoga/eight-limbs-of-yoga.

258. **reduction in postpartum depression:** Melissa M. Buttner et al., "Efficacy of Yoga for Depressed Postpartum Women: A Randomized Controlled Trial," *Complementary Therapies in Clinical Practice* 21, no. 2 (2015): 94–100, https://doi.org/10.1016/j.ctcp.2015.03.003.

259. **no need for *mula bandha*:** Courtney Sullivan, "How to Work Your Pelvic Floor with Mula Bandha," Healthline, April 23, 2020, https://www.healthline.com/health/overactive-bladder/pelvic-floor-with-mula-bandha#1.

Chapter 13. Pilates

269. **quality of postpartum sleep:** Farzaneh Ashrafinia et al., "The Effects of Pilates Exercise on Sleep Quality in Postpartum Women," *Journal of Bodywork and Movement Therapies* 18, no. 2 (2013): 190–99, https://doi.org/10.1016/j.jbmt.2013.09.007.

269. **and increase energy:** Karl M. Fleming and Matthew P. Herring, "The Effects of Pilates on Mental Health Outcomes: A Meta-Analysis of Controlled Trials," *Complementary Therapies in Medicine* 37 (2018): 80–95, https://doi.org/10.1016/j.ctim.2018.02.003.

270. **avulsion of the pelvic floor:** Lauren N. Siff et al., "The Effect of Commonly Performed Exercises on the Levator Hiatus Area and the Length and Strength of Pelvic Floor Muscles in Postpartum Women," *Female Pelvic Medicine & Reconstructive Surgery* 26, no. 1 (2020): 61–66, https://doi.org/10.1097/spv.0000000000000590.

270. **Michael King recommends:** Michael King and Yolande Green, *Pilates Workbook for Pregnancy: Illustrated Step-by-Step Matwork Techniques* (Berkeley, CA: Ulysses Press, 2002).

278. **prone to stress urinary incontinence (SUI):** Liga Blyholder et al., "Exercise Behaviors and Health Conditions of Runners After Childbirth," *Sports Health: A Multidisciplinary Approach* 9, no. 1 (2016): 45–51, https://doi.org/10.1177/1941738116673605.

278. **running-related injury:** Shefali M. Christopher et al., "Common Musculoskeletal Impairments in Postpartum Runners: An International Delphi Study," *Archives of Physiotherapy* 10 (2020): article 19, https://doi.org/10.1186/s40945-020-00090-y.

278. **odds of leaking:** Isabel S. Moore et al., "Multidisciplinary, Biopsychosocial Factors Contributing to Return to Running and Running Related Stress Urinary Incontinence in Postpartum Women," *British Journal of Sports Medicine* 55, no. 22 (2021): 1286–92, https://doi.org/10.1136/bjsports-2021-104168.

282. **pain or leakage:** Rachel Selman et al., "Maximizing Recovery in the Postpartum Period: A Timeline for Rehabilitation from Pregnancy through Return to Sport," *International Journal of Sports Physical Therapy* 17, no. 6 (2022): 1170–83, https://doi.org/10.26603/001c.37863.

Chapter 15. Kettlebell

286. **reduced symptoms of depression and anxiety:** Weverton Rufo-Tavares et al., "Effects of Kettlebell Training and Detraining on Mood Status and Sleep and Life Quality of Healthy Women," *Journal of Bodywork and Movement Therapies* 24, no. 4 (2020): 344–53, https://doi.org/10.1016/j.jbmt.2020.07.006.

INDEX

ABOUT THE AUTHORS

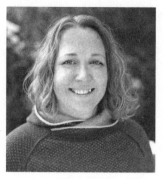 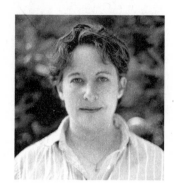

Photographs of the authors © William Trevaskis

Ruth E. Macy, PT, DPT, is a pelvic floor physical therapist with seventeen years of experience in the field. She is passionate about working with people to achieve their desired health outcomes, removing bias and exclusion in healthcare, and delivering a compassionate patient-centered approach that eliminates shame and blame in the ownership of the human body. When she's not at work, she enjoys smashing the patriarchy, paddleboarding, spoiling her dog, and winning at board games with her family.

Courtney Naliboff is a teacher, writer, musician, volunteer EMT, parent, and swimming enthusiast who lives on North Haven, a tiny unbridged island off of Maine's Midcoast, with her husband and daughter. She is a longtime reporter and columnist for *The Working Waterfront* and has written about Jewish parenting in small-town Maine for *Kveller*, *Hey Alma*, and *The Bangor Daily News*.